MCQs for the MRCP
Part 1–Paediatrics

N. G. Barakat MBBCh, MRCP(UK)
Child Health Department,
St. George's Hospital Medical School
London

M. O'Callaghan MBBS, MRCP(UK)
Consultant Paediatrician,
Whipp's Cross Hospital
London

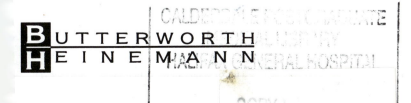

BUTTERWORTH
HEINEMANN

To our parents and families

Butterworth-Heinemann Ltd
Linacre House, Jordan Hill, Oxford OX2 8DP

R̵ A member of the Reed Elsevier plc group

OXFORD LONDON BOSTON
MUNICH NEW DELHI SINGAPORE SYDNEY
TOKYO TORONTO WELLINGTON

First published 1994

© Butterworth-Heinemann Ltd 1994

British Library Cataloguing in Publication Data
Barakat, N. G.
  MCQs for the MRCP Part 1–Paediatrics
  I. Title II. O'Callaghan, M.
  618.920076

ISBN 0 7506 2029 3

Typeset by TecSet Ltd, Wallington, Surrey
Printed and bound in Great Britain by Biddles Ltd, Guildford and King's Lynn

Contents

Preface

The paediatric option of the MRCP (UK) Part 1 examination was first introduced in October 1993 necessitating an MCQ book focussing more specifically on paediatric topics. Each chapter in this book contains questions designed to test candidates' knowledge of the basic sciences as well as clinical conditions. Areas covered include molecular biology, biochemistry, physiology, microbiology, pathology, immunology, pharmacology and statistics.

We wish to thank all our colleagues, former teachers and examiners who have unwittingly provided ideas for many of the questions. In addition Ms Lobna Maktari and Mrs Shirley Miller have provided a great deal of support and help in the preparation of this text.

MO'C
NB

The MRCP Part 1 examination

The paediatric option of the MRCP Part 1 examination was first introduced in October 1993. The paediatric and general medicine options share approximately 50% of questions which cover areas of equal relevance to both groups of candidates. There is an increasing emphasis on basic science topics in the Part 1 examination. Both options have the same pass rate. The top 35% of candidates will pass the examination which means that the actual pass mark varies, but is usually around 55–60%.

The actual examination is a multiple choice question paper consisting of 60 questions. The multiple choice questions are designed to test the candidates' reasoning ability as well as their knowledge of basic facts. Each question consists of a stem statement with five following items. The candidate has to answer each item as 'true', 'false', or 'don't know'. It is important to read the stem and items carefully, but answer each item independently disregarding the other statements in the question. The answer sheets are read by an automatic document reader so mark the answer paper boldly and clearly. If you change your answer erase it carefully and re-mark the paper.

On your first run through of the examination paper either mark the answers in the question paper or straight onto the answer sheet. Leave enough time at the end to go over your answers and check that the answer sheet is correctly marked. Try again to answer any difficult questions but avoid repeated reviews as this is usually counter-productive.

The examination is negatively marked which means that one mark is deducted for each incorrect answer. The pass mark will vary but in general aim to answer a minimum of 250 questions.

Preparing for the examination

It is important to achieve a good knowledge of the basic sciences relevant to clinical paediatrics. The recommended texts are useful, but also try to attend a course specifically designed for the paediatric Part 1 examination. Once you have acquired the basic knowledge start to do MCQs, the results of which will give you a guide to any gaps in your knowledge. Do as many MCQs as possible aiming to score over 60% correct.

MCQ examination technique

It is important to accept the questions at face value and not to look for hidden meanings or ambiguities. Try to avoid genuine guessing but at the same time do not give in too easily and try to reason through the question without spending too long on the problem. If you are 'fairly certain' of the answer commit yourself on the answer sheet rather than recording a 'don't know'.

The wording of MCQs may present some difficulty and the meaning of many terms is outlined in the following table. Be wary of universal statements such as 'only', 'never', 'invariable' and 'always' which are usually false.

Terminology used in MCQs

Always	There are no recognized exceptions
Never	
Can Be	Reported (or recognized) to occur
May be	
Occurs	No statement of frequency
Commonly	An occurrence rate of greater than 50%
Frequently	
Likely	
Often	
Characteristic	Features which occur frequently enough to be of
Typical	diagnostic significance although they are not pathognomonic
Specific	A feature that occurs only in the named disease and
Pathognomonic	no other
Recognized feature	It has been reported to be a feature or association

In summary the best preparation for the examination is a combination of knowledge and plenty of MCQ practice including past papers. If you are well prepared you are likely to pass, but remember that most members of the Royal College of Physicians will have failed some part of the exam on at least one occasion.

Recommended texts and references

W.F. Ganong (1991) *Review of Medical Physiology*, 15th edn. Appleton and Lange

J. Widdicombe and A. Davies (1983) *Respiratory Physiology*, 2nd edn. Edward Arnold

J. Mcleod, C. Edwards and I. Bouchier (1992) *Davidson's Principles of Medicine*, 16th edn. Churchill Livingstone

A.G.M. Campbell and N. McIntosh (1992) *Forfar Textbook of Paediatrics*, 4th edn. Churchill Livingstone

R.E. Behrman, R.M. Kleigman, W.E. Nelson and V.C. Vaughan (1992) *Nelson's Textbook of Paediatrics*, 14th edn. Saunders

T.J. David (1991, 1992) *Recent Advances in Paediatrics*, Vols 9 and 10. Churchill Livingstone

R.S. Illingworth (1987) *The Development of Infants and Young Children*, 9th edn. Churchill Livingstone

C.P. Wendall Smith, P.L. Williams and A.Treadgold (1984) *Basic Human Embryology*, 3rd edn. Pitman

D.R. Laurence, P.N. Bennett, and P. Kneebone (1987) *Clinical Pharmacology*, 6th edn. Churchill Livingstone

R.M. Reece (1987) *Manual of Emergency Paediatrics*, 3rd edn. Saunders

Embryology

1. **The following statements relating to gametogenesis are correct**
   a. Chromosomes are reduced from diploid to haploid numbers by meiotic division
   b. Chromosome pairs are usually in close proximity to each other
   c. During prophase the chromosomes become longer and thinner
   d. During metaphase the chromosomes line-up in the linear plane
   e. Division of cytoplasm occurs during telophase

2. **The female sexual cycle is controlled by the following hormones**
   a. Gonadotrophic releasing hormones
   b. Follicular stimulating hormones
   c. Lutenizing hormones
   d. Oestrogens
   e. Testosterone

3. **Fertilization**
   a. Occurs in the body of uterus
   b. Results in the restoration of the haploid number of chromosomes
   c. The sex of the foetus is determined by the XX chromosomes on the ova
   d. Is followed immediately by secondary meiotic division
   e. Occurs when the sperm penetrates the oocyte cell membrane

4. **True or false**
   a. By the 8th day post-fertilization, the trophoblast appears as a large mononuclear cell
   b. The embryonic period extends from the 3rd–11th weeks of gestation
   c. Implantation usually occurs within 72 hours post-fertilization
   d. The three germ cell layers start to appear by the end of the 5th week of gestation
   e. Neural-plate is formed from the ectodermal germ layer

Answers overleaf

1. a. True
    b. False   They are only close to each other only during the meiotic or maturation division of germ cells
    c. False   They will continue to condense and become shorter and thicker
    d. False   They line-up in the equatorial plane
    e. True

2. a. True
    b. True
    c. True
    d. False
    e. False

3. a. False   Ampullary region of the uterine tube
    b. False   Diploid
    c. False   By the Y chromosome on the spermatazoa
    d. True
    e. True   And crosses the zona pellucida

4. a. True   The syncytiotrophoblast is characterized by an outer multinucleated zone without distinct cell boundaries
    b. False   From the 3rd–8th weeks of gestation
    c. False   Usually occurs in the first week post-fertilization
    d. False   By the 3rd week of gestation at the same time as the mesodermal and ectodermal germ cell layers
    e. True

5. **The following systems or organs are derived from the mesodermal germ cell layer**
a. Blood
b. Lenses
c. Dermis
d. Spleen
e. Vitellin duct

6. **The following agents can cause damage during the embryonic period**
a. The Rubella virus
b. Trimethadone
c. Diethyl stillboestrol
d. Vitamin A
e. Hyperthermia

7. **The following drugs may cause congenital abnormalities if they are taken by the mother during pregnancy**
a. Lithium
b. Chloramphenicol
c. Phenytoin
d. Warfarin
e. Atropine

8. **The following statements relating to the development of the foetal respiratory system are correct**
a. The muscular component arises from the mesodermal germ cell layer
b. By 7 weeks' gestation gas exchange by the alveoli is possible
c. Surfactant is produced by the alveolar type I epithelial cells
d. The growth of the lungs is measured by the increase in the size of the alveoli
e. Alveolar formation stops after the foetal period

Answers overleaf

5. a. True   And blood vessels and other vascular elements
   b. False   Develops from ectoderm
   c. True   As well as the subcutaneous tissue of the skin
   d. True
   e. False   From the endodermal germ cell layer

6. a. True
   b. True   Can cause cardiac malformations, cleft palate, urogenital and skeletal abnormalities
   c. True   Vaginal cancer and maldescended testes
   d. True   Heart defects, and cleft-palate and lip
   e. False

7. a. True   Heart defects (Ebstein anomaly)
   b. False
   c. True   Facial defects and mental retardation
   d. True   Chondrodysplasia and microcephaly
   e. False

8. a. True
   b. True
   c. False   From type II alveolar epithelial cells
   d. False   The size of the lungs increases due to the formation of additional respiratory bronchioles and alveoli
   e. False   Formation of new alveoli occurs for the first few years of postnatal life

9. **Development of the foetal digestive system is characterized by**
   a. The lining epithelium of the gastrointestinal tract is derived from the mesodermal germ cell layer
   b. The foregut gives rise to the pancreas
   c. Physiological herniation of the midgut occurs at the age of 12 weeks gestation
   d. The failure of the midgut to rotate through 270° counter-clockwise can lead to malrotation
   e. Distal parts of the rectum and anus arise from the ectodermal germ cell layer

10. **The following statements about the development of the foetal urogenital system are correct**
    a. Failure to connect between the collecting and excretory system can lead to cyst formation
    b. Early division of the ureteric buds results in a duplex system
    c. The Y-chromosome causes failure of the cortical (ovarian) cord to develop
    d. Testosterone stimulates the development of the external genitalia
    e. The mesonephron will form the excretory system

Answers overleaf

9. a. False   From the endodermal germ cell layer. Muscular and peritoneal components arise from the mesodermal germ cell layer

    b. True   And also the stomach, duodenum, liver, peritoneum and biliary system

    c. False   Usually at the age of 6 weeks

    d. True   As well as stenosis and duplication of the intestinal tract

    e. True

10. a. True   And renal agenesis

    b. True

    c. True   As well as the development of the medullary cord (testes) and formation of the tunica albuginea

    d. False   Dihydrocortisone is responsible for formation of the external genitalia in males, while testosterone stimulates the mesonephric ducts (vas deferens and epididymis)

    e. True

Neonatology

1. **True or false**
   a. The Perinatal Mortality Rate (PMR) is the number of stillbirths and deaths in the first week of life per 1000 live births
   b. The Infant Mortality Rate (IMR) is the number of deaths under the age of 6 months per 1000 live births
   c. The Neonatal Mortality Rate (NMR) is the number of deaths from 0–28 days per 1000 live births
   d. The stillbirth rate is the number of deaths per 1000 births
   e. The Postnatal Mortality Rate (PMR) is the deaths from 1–11 years of age per 1000 live births

2. **Characteristic features of Erb's palsy include**
   a. A lesion of C5 and 6
   b. Paralysis of the deltoid and brachioradialis muscles
   c. Abnormal grasp reflex
   d. Biceps and Moro reflexes are absent on the affected side
   e. Respiratory distress may be the presenting feature

3. **The following statements relating to jaundice extending beyond the first 14 days of life are correct**
   a. Acholic stool is a feature of biliary atresia
   b. Kasai's portoentrostomy is the commonest operation for biliary atresia
   c. Infants with biliary atresia operated on in the first 2 months of life have a 90% chance of survival
   d. Physiological jaundice usually persists beyond 14 days of age
   e. The 5 year survival rate after Kasai's operation at the age of 6 months is 50–60%

4. **Complications of parenteral feeding in premature babies include**
   a. Necrotizing enterocolitis
   b. Cholestasis
   c. Hyperglycaemia
   d. Respiratory failure
   e. Sepsis

Answers overleaf

11

1. a. True
   b. False   IMR is the number of deaths below one year of age per 1000 live births
   c. False   NMR is the number of deaths from 7–28 days of age per 1000 live births
   d. True
   e. False   PMR is the number of deaths from 1–11 months of age per 1000 live births

2. a. True   May extend to affect C4 and lead to respiratory distress
   b. True   Biceps is also affected
   c. False   Normal grasp reflex as the small muscles of the hand are not affected
   d. True
   e. True

3. a. True
   b. True   And should be performed before 2 months of age
   c. True
   d. False
   e. False   Only if it is carried out before the age of 3 months.

4. a. False   Early oral feeding can cause NEC in preterm babies
   b. True   This is due to immaturity of the liver enzymes
   c. True
   d. False
   e. True

5. **Characteristic features of respiratory distress syndrome include**
   a. Tachypnoea
   b. Inspiratory grunting
   c. Sternal and intercostal recession
   d. Peripheral cyanosis alone
   e. Air bronchogram on CXR

6. **The following statements relating to the pathophysiology of RDS are correct**
   a. There is increased lung compliance
   b. A right to left shunt occurs in up to 70% of cases through a patent ductus arteriosus
   c. 2.3 DPG levels are low
   d. Lung volume is reduced
   e. There is hypoxia with a low pH

7. **Recognized complications of surfactant therapy in RDS include**
   a. Pulmonary haemorrhage
   b. An increased incidence of of broncho-pulmonary dysplasia (BPD)
   c. An increased incidence of patent ductus arteriosus
   d. An increase in O_2 requirements
   e. Infection

8. **Common causes of congenital pneumonia include**
   a. Group B beta haemolytic streptococci
   b. Respiratory syncitial virus (RSV)
   c. Listeria monocytogenes
   d. Staphylococcus aureus
   e. Herpes simplex virus

9. **Complications of RDS or its therapy include**
   a. Pneumothorax
   b. Pulmonary interstitial emphysema (PIE) in 25% of patients
   c. Intraventricular haemorrhage (IVH)
   d. Broncho-pulmonary dysplasia (BPD)
   e. Pneumopericardium

Answers overleaf

5. a. True
   b. False
   c. True
   d. False
   e. True   Characteristic features of RDS are: expiratory grunting, cyanosis, intercostal and subcostal recession, tachypnoea, ground glass appearance and air bronchogram on CXR

6. a. False   Lung compliance decreases as the lungs becomes stiff with reduced tissue elasticity
   b. False
   c. False
   d. False   Lung volume is increased with hyperinflation
   e. True   And high P_{CO_2} (metabolic and respiratory acidosis)

7. a. True
   b. False   Incidence of BPD is reduced with surfactant treatment
   c. True
   d. False
   e. False

8. a. True
   b. False   Respiratory syncitial virus can be acquired postnatally
   c. True
   d. False   Not common
   e. False   Not common

9. a. True
   b. False   The overall incidence is $< 25\%$
   c. True
   d. True
   e. True   Not common but occurs in 1.6% of infants with RDS

10. **The following statements relating to congenital abnormalities of the lungs are correct**
    a. Potter's syndrome is associated with pulmonary hypoplasia
    b. Congenital lobar emphysema usually affects the right upper lobe
    c. Cystic adenomatoid malformations of the lung cannot be diagnosed antenatally
    d. Laryngomalacia with stridor may present on the first day of life
    e. Tracheo-oesophageal fistula may present with choking

11. **Interstitial pneumonitis in newborn infants can be caused by the following infections**
    a. Cytomegalovirus (CMV)
    b. Respiratory synctial virus (RSV)
    c. Chlamydia
    d. Adenovirus
    e. Varicella zoster

12. **Complications found more commonly in SGA (small for gestational age) infants than post-term infants include**
    a. Meconium aspiration syndrome
    b. Pulmonary haemorrhage
    c. Necrotizing enterocolitis
    d. Hypocalcaemia
    e. Rickets

13. **Aetiological factors associated with preterm labour include**
    a. A higher incidence in social class I
    b. Smoking
    c. Maternal diabetes mellitus
    d. Maternal tuberculosis infection
    e. Intrauterine infection

Answers overleaf

10. a. True
    b. False Congenital lobar emphysema is commonest in the left lower lobe
    c. False Can be diagnosed antenatally by US
    d. True
    e. True

11. a. True
    b. True
    c. True
    d. True
    e. True

12. a. False Meconium aspiration can be associated with both
    b. True
    c. True   Necrotizing enterocolitis is most commonly associated with preterm infants
    d. True
    e. False Rickets is commonly associated with prematurity

13. a. False Most frequent in social classes IV and V
    b. False Smoking may cause SGA
    c. True
    d. True
    e. True

14. **Congenital heart defects which may present early with heart failure in newborn infants include**
    a. Hypoplastic left heart syndrome
    b. Tetralogy of Fallot
    c. Severe coarctation of the aorta
    d. Patent ductus arteriosus (PDA)
    e. Ventricular septal defect (VSD)

15. **Factors known to precipitate necrotising enterocolitis (NEC) include**
    a. Early feeding in preterm infants
    b. Polycythaemia
    c. Breast milk
    d. Umbilical catheterization
    e. Perinatal asphyxia

16. **Diagnostic features of NEC include**
    a. Distended abdomen
    b. Tenderness and guarding
    c. Intramural gas on abdominal X-ray
    d. Subdiaphragmatic air
    e. Oedema of the abdominal wall

17. **Causes of jaundice in the first 24 hours of life include**
    a. A glucose-6-phosphate dehydrogenase deficiency
    b. Prematurity
    c. Physiological jaundice
    d. ABO incompatibility
    e. Sepsis

18. **Known complications of exchange transfusion include**
    a. Cytomegalovirus (CMV) infection
    b. Hyperkalaemia
    c. Hypercalcaemia
    d. Hypothermia
    e. Alkalosis

Answers overleaf

14. a. True
    b. False
    c. True
    d. True
    e. True

15. a. True   Formula milk feeding
    b. True
    c. False   Breast feeding provides partial protection against NEC
    d. True
    e. True

16. a. False
    b. False
    c. True
    d. False   This occurs with intestinal perforation
    e. True

17. a. True
    b. False   This usually starts after the first 24 hours of life
    c. False   Usually after 24 hours
    d. True   Also rhesus isoimmune haemolytic anaemia, sepsis, hereditary spherocytosis and galactosaemia
    e. True

18. a. True   Early complications of exchange transfusions include: hyperkalaemia, hypoglycaemia, acidosis, hypocalcaemia, hypothermia. Late complications include: anaemia, cholestasis, portal vein thrombosis and alkalosis
    b. True
    c. False
    d. True   If babies are left exposed
    e. True

19. Polycythaemia in newborn infants can be due to
a. Intra-uterine growth retardation (IUGR)
b. Cyanotic congenital heart disease
c. Post-maturity
d. Down's syndrome
e. Twin-to-twin transfusion

20. Maternal drugs which cause thrombocytopenia in newborn infants include
a. Chlorothiazide
b. Digoxin
c. Erythromycin
d. Phenylbutazone
e. Indomethacin

21. Factors which lower vitamin K levels in newborn babies include
a. Breast feeding
b. Bacterial over-growth in the intestine
c. Cephalosporins
d. Maternal anti-convulsants
e. Vitamin E

22. The following statements relating to neonatal meningitis are correct
a. *E. coli* is a common causative organism
b. Lethargy and apnoea are characteristic features
c. Cefotaxime plus ampicillin can be used as treatment
d. May follow urinary tract infection
e. Neurodevelopmental complications occur in a third of survivors

23. Post haemorrhagic hydrocephalus
a. Does not usually require shunting
b. Has a worse prognosis than congenital hydrocephalus
c. More than two-thirds of affected patients will have normal intelligence
d. Acetazolamide can be used in the treatment
e. Is usually non communicating

Answers overleaf

19. a. True
    b. False   This occurs later
    c. True
    d. True
    e. True   The mortality is higher in the polycythaemic twin

20. a. True
    b. True
    c. False
    d. True
    e. True   Causes of thrombocytopenia other than drugs include: infections (congenital or acquired), asphyxia, acidosis and maternal antibodies (ITP, SLE)

21. a. True   Human milk contains low levels of Vitamin K when compared with cow's milk
    b. False
    c. True   Prevents bacterial growth
    d. True
    e. False

22. a. True
    b. False   These are non-specific clinical signs
    c. True
    d. True
    e. True   Deafness is the commonest followed by behaviour and learning problems.

23. a. True
    b. True
    c. False
    d. True
    e. False   Is usually communicating hydrocephalus

24. **The following features are associated with specific congenital renal abnormalities**
    a. Infantile polycystic kidney — hepatic fibrosis
    b. Bilateral renal agenesis — Potter's syndrome
    c. Horse shoe kidney — renal failure
    d. Posterior urethral valves — poor urinary stream
    e. Ectopic kidneys — hypertension

25. **Early neonatal hypocalcaemia may be due to**
    a. Low birth weight (LBW)
    b. Intra-uterine growth retardation
    c. Asphyxia
    d. Infants of diabetic mothers
    e. Alkalosis

26. **Features more suggestive of congenital rubella syndrome than congenital toxoplasmosis are**
    a. Macrocephaly
    b. Cataracts
    c. Hepatosplenomegaly
    d. Microphthalmia
    e. Patent ductus arteriosus (PDA)

27. **Features suggestive of congenital CMV infection rather than toxoplasmosis include**
    a. Periventricular calcification
    b. Chorioretinitis
    c. Microcephaly
    d. Sensorineural deafness
    e. Intrauterine growth retardation (IUGR)

Answers overleaf

24. a. True
 b. True Features of Potter's syndrome include abnormal facies, hypoplastic lungs, cardiac and skeletal anomalies
 c. False Normal renal function
 d. True
 e. True

25. a. True
 b. True
 c. True
 d. True
 e. True

26. a. False Microcephaly is usually a feature of congenital rubella syndrome
 b. True
 c. False
 d. False In both
 e. True

27. a. True Other features of congenital CMV infection include: microcephaly, deafness, IUGR, chorioretinitis, purpura, jaundice, microphthalmia, haemolytic anaemia, pneumonitis
 b. False
 c. True
 d. False
 e. False

28. **The following statements relating to neonatal chickenpox infection are correct**
    a. Zoster immunoglobulin prevents the infection
    b. Babies whose mothers develop the chickenpox rash upto and including 5 days before delivery should receive zoster immunoglobulin
    c. Babies whose mother develop the chickenpox rash upto 5 days after delivery should receive zoster immunoglobulin
    d. Gancyclovir is the treatment of choice for neonatal varicella-zoster infection
    e. The mortality rate is < 10% if babies develop chickenpox within 5 days of birth

29. **Aetiological factors responsible for transient hypoglycaemia with normal plasma insulin levels in newborn infants include**
    a. Intra-uterine growth retardation
    b. Congenital heart disease
    c. Infants of diabetic mothers
    d. Nesidioblastosis
    e. Inborn errors of metabolism

30. **Common and late manifestations of congenital rubella infection include**
    a. Interstitial pneumonitis
    b. Diabetes mellitus
    c. Cataracts
    d. Retinopathy
    e. Autism

Answers overleaf

28. a. False   It ameliorates the infection
     b. True
     c. True
     d. False   Acyclovir
     e. False   Up to 30% will die if a rash develops 5–10 days after birth

29. a. True
     b. True
     c. False   Insulin levels are high
     d. False   Persistent hypoglycaemia with high insulin levels
     e. True   As well as persistent hypoglycaemia with normal or low insulin levels

30. a. True
     b. False
     c. True
     d. True
     e. False

Genetics

1. **Deoxyribonucleic acid (DNA) is characterized by the following features**
   a. A polynucleotide chain with a single helix
   b. Nitrogenous bases as part of its composition
   c. Guanine always pairs with thymine
   d. Genetic information is stored in the form of triplet codes
   e. It is mainly found in the nucleolus of cells

2. **The following statements relating to ribonucleic acid (RNA) are correct**
   a. The adenine base of DNA is replaced by uracil in RNA
   b. mRNA is synthesized in the nucleus
   c. tRNA is mainly found in the cytoplasmic reticulum
   d. The RNA-polymerase enzyme copies one strand of DNA to single stranded RNA
   e. Ribosomes are the site of protein synthesis

3. **Gastro-intestinal tract abnormalities associated with Down's syndrome include**
   a. Imperforate anus
   b. Pyloric stenosis
   c. Hirschsprung's disease
   d. Oesophageal atresia
   e. Duodenal atresia

4. **Systemic diseases which have an increased incidence in Down's syndrome include**
   a. Hyperthyroidism
   b. Acute lymphoblastic leukaemia
   c. Diabetes mellitus
   d. Alzheimer's disease
   e. Eissenmenger's syndrome

Answers overleaf

1. a. False   It is a double helix
   b. True   Purines which are adenine and guanine and
                  pyrimidines which are cytosine and thymine
   c. False   Guanine with cytosine and adenine with thymine
   d. True
   e. False   Is usually in the chromosomes

2. a. False   Thymine replaced by uracil
   b. True
   c. False   In the cytoplasm
   d. True
   e. True

3. a. True
   b. False   Duodenal atresia and other intestinal atresias are
                  common
   c. True
   d. True
   e. True

4. a. False   Hypothyroidism
   b. True
   c. True
   d. True
   e. True   Due to cyanotic congenital heart disease

5. X-linked recessive inheritance is characterized by
   a. All daughters of an affected father will be affected
   b. Males are more severely affected than females
   c. All daughters of an affected male are carriers
   d. All sons of a carrier mother are affected
   e. A female carrier has a 25% chance of having an affected son

6. Syndromes associated with chromosomal abnormalities include
   a. Cri du-chat — deletion of 5p
   b. Klinefelter's — 47 XYY
   c. Noonan's syndrome — 45 OX
   d. Edward's syndrome — Trisomy 13
   e. Retinoblastoma — abnormality of chromosome 13

7. Features of Turner's syndrome include
   a. Short stature
   b. Aortic stenosis
   c. A 30% risk of mental retardation
   d. Alopecia
   e. Deafness in 30% of cases

8. Syndromes associated with microcephaly include
   a. Rubella syndrome
   b. Cornelia De-Lange
   c. Sotos syndrome
   d. Belephrophimosis
   e. Apert's syndrome

Answers overleaf

5. a. False   X-linked dominant disorders
    b. True
    c. True
    d. False   Only 50% chance of inheriting the disease
    e. True

6. a. True
    b. False   47 XXY
    c. False   Normal chromosomal numbers. 45 XO associated with Turner's syndrome
    d. False   Trisomy 18
    e. False   Chromosome 11

7. a. True
    b. True   Coarctation of the aorta is the commonest congenital cardiac defect
    c. False   Less than 15% of cases
    d. False
    e. True   And recurrent otitis media in more than 60% of cases

8. a. True
    b. True   Mental and growth retardation, bushy eye lashes, synophrus, long philtrum and congenital heart lesions
    c. False   Tall stature and a large head with mental retardation
    d. False
    e. False   Acrocephaly and syndactyly of all fingers with mental retardation are other features

9. **Laxity of joints is a feature of**
   a. Ehler–Danlos syndrome
   b. Down's syndrome
   c. Osteogenesis imperfecta
   d. Aarskog's syndrome
   e. Arthrogryposis multiplexa

10. **Deafness is a common feature of**
   a. Treacher–Collins syndrome
   b. Refsum's syndrome
   c. Waardenburg's syndrome
   d. Hurler's syndrome
   e. Neurofibromatosis type I

11. **Common congenital causes of cataracts include**
   a. Galactosaemia
   b. Incontentia pigmenti
   c. Dystrophia myotonica
   d. Lowe's syndrome
   e. Hypoparathyroidism

12. **Characteristic features of Noonan's syndrome include**
   a. Autosomal recessive inheritance
   b. Atrial septal defect
   c. Ptosis
   d. Short stature
   e. Elfin facies

Answers overleaf

9. a. True   Increased skin laxity, cigarette paper scars and fragile blood vessels are other features

     b. False   Associated with hypotonia

     c. True   Fragile bones with repeated fractures, otosclerosis and odontosclerosis imperfecta

     d. True   Short stature, empty scrotum, and small penis are other features

     e. False   Stiffness of joints is a common feature

10. a. True   Autosomal dominant inheritance with mandibulofacial dysostosis and microtia with absent external auditory canal

     b. False   Ataxia, ichthyosis, retinitis pigmentosa, peripheral neuropathy with raised serum phytanic and fatty acid levels

     c. True   Heterochromia of the iris and a white forelock

     d. True

     e. False   Type-II is associated with acoustic neuromas

11. a. True

     b. False

     c. True

     d. True   Buphthalmos and mental retardation are other features

     e. False

12. a. False   Mental retardation is common. Pulmonary stenosis and cardiac septal hypertrophy are other cardiac features

     b. True

     c. True

     d. True   Female is usually fertile

     e. False   This is a feature of William's syndrome

13. Characteristic features of William's syndrome include
   a. Moderate mental retardation
   b. Webbed neck
   c. Thick lips
   d. Long philtrum
   e. Hypercalcaemia

14. The following conditions are inherited in an autosomal dominant fashion
   a. Poland syndrome
   b. Tuberose sclerosis
   c. Anglemann's syndrome
   d. Ornithine carbamyl transferase deficiency
   e. Laurence–Moon–Biedle syndrome

15. Autosomal recessive inheritance disorders include
   a. Aarskog's syndrome
   b. Russell–Silver syndrome
   c. Thanotrophic dwarfism
   d. Albinism
   e. Becker muscular dystrophy

Answers overleaf

13. a. True   As well as prominent lips and anteverted nares
     b. False   This is a feature of Noonan's syndrome
     c. True   And dysphonia
     d. False   Not characteristic
     e. True   Supra-aortic stenosis is another feature

14. a. False   Sporadic
     b. True
     c. False   Sporadic
     d. False   X-linked dominant
     e. False   Autosomal recessive

15. a. False   X-linked disorder
     b. False   Sporadic
     c. True   And may also be dominantly inherited
     d. True
     e. False   X-linked recessive

Nutrition

1. **Drugs contraindicated during breast feeding include**
   a. Cimetidine
   b. Metronidazole
   c. Digoxin
   d. Tetracycline
   e. Bromocriptine

2. **The following statements relating to carbohydrate metabolism in children are correct**
   a. Glucose is broken down into pyruvic acid by the anaerobic pathway (glycolysis)
   b. Disaccharides are absorbed in the membrane fraction of the microvilli
   c. Galactose is hydrolysed to give two glucose molecules
   d. Most of the absorbed sugar is converted to glycogen in the liver
   e. Fructose is actively taken up against a concentration gradient in the small intestine

3. **Vitamin K deficiency may be due to**
   a. Anti-convulsant drugs
   b. Antibiotics
   c. Biliary obstruction
   d. Prematurity
   e. Breast feeding

4. **Deficiency of the following vitamins can lead to the associated abnormalities**
   a. Vitamin E — haemolysis in preterm babies
   b. Vitamin C — poor wound healing
   c. Biotin — dermatitis
   d. Thiamine — pellagra
   e. Vitamin A — nyctolopia

Answers overleaf

1. a. False
   b. False Should be avoided if possible
   c. False Is a safe drug
   d. True   As it can cause staining of teeth
   e. True

2. a. True   And to water and carbon dioxide by the
               tricarboxylic acid cycle
   b. False Disaccharides are absorbed at the brush border
               while disaccharidase hydrolyses disaccharides to
               monosaccharides in the membrane fraction of the
               microvilli
   c. False Lactose is hydrolysed to glucose and galactose,
               sucrose is hydrolysed to glucose and fructose,
               maltose is hydrolysed to two glucose molecules
   d. True
   e. False Fructose is taken up by passive transport

3. a. True
   b. True   Antibiotics kill the producers of vitamin K in the
               intestine (bacteria)
   c. True   As it is fat soluble
   d. True
   e. True   Has a low concentration of vitamin K

4. a. True
   b. True   And purpuric-like rash
   c. True   And dementia
   d. False Thiamine deficiency can lead to beriberi and
               niacin deficiency to pellagra
   e. True   Plus keratomalacia, photophobia and
               xerophthalmia. It is the commonest cause of
               blindness in the third world

5. The following substances are found in higher concentrations in formula than breast milk
   a. Sodium
   b. Polyunsaturated fatty acids
   c. Casein
   d. Phenylalanine
   e. Lactose

6. The following statements relating to vitamin A deficiency are correct
   a. Osteoporosis may occur
   b. Xerophthalmia is common
   c. Corneal perforation is common
   d. Complications are not completely curable with vitamin A treatment
   e. It is associated with steatorrhoea

7. The following statements relating to essential fatty acids are correct
   a. Linolenic acid is the precursor of prostaglandin
   b. Linolenic acid is essential for normal neurological functioning
   c. Both linolenic and linoleic acid are synthesized by humans
   d. Excess of essential fatty acids can cause desquamation of the skin
   e. Unsaturated fatty acids are necessary for the normal growth of hair and skin

8. Features of pyridoxine deficiency (vitamin B_6) include
   a. Stomatitis
   b. Megaloblastic anaemia
   c. May occur following anti-tuberculous therapy
   d. Increased xanthurenic acid levels
   e. Seizures

Answers overleaf

5. a. True
    b. False   More in breast milk
    c. True   Vitamins found in higher concentrations in breast milk include vitamins D and C
    d. True
    e. False   More in breast milk

6. a. False   This may occur if there is an excess of vitamin A
    b. True
    c. False   It is rare and occurs only in untreated cases
    d. False   Complete response is common
    e. False   It is a water soluble vitamin

7. a. True   Linolenic is the precursor of prostaglandins, arachodinic acid and leukotrienes
    b. True
    c. False   They are not synthesized by humans and need to be supplied through food
    d. False   Decrease in essential fatty acid can cause skin desquamation
    e. True

8. a. False   Occurs with vitamin B_{12} deficiency
    b. False   Vitamin B_{12} and folic acid deficiency are the main causes
    c. True   Isoniazid is a liver enzyme inducer
    d. True
    e. True

Growth, development and puberty

1. **Primitive reflexes disappear at the following ages**
   a. Moro reflex — 6–7 months
   b. Grasp reflex—2–3 months
   c. Placing response — 6 months
   d. Walking reflex — 10–12 weeks
   e. Tonic neck reflex — 2–3 months

2. **The following reflexes appear later as the infant develops**
   a. Body righting at 3 months
   b. Abdominal reflex at 6 months
   c. Landau at 3 months
   d. Parachute at 9 months
   e. Tendon reflexes at 3–6 months

3. **Infants at the age of 6 months can be expected to**
   a. Sit with their head held up
   b. Take weight on their feet
   c. Transfer objects from one hand to another
   d. Look for hidden objects
   e. Feed themselves crackers

4. **At the age of 12 months, the infant**
   a. Can stand from a sitting position
   b. Can drop and throw toys
   c. Can stand alone
   d. Knows his name and the time
   e. Plays pat-a-cake

5. **A 2-year-old child can be expected to**
   a. Run
   b. Turn single pages in a book
   c. Use thread and beads
   d. Ask for the toilet as needed
   e. Use 200 recognisable words

Answers overleaf

1. a. False   At 3–4 months
    b. True
    c. False   At 3 months of age
    d. False   At 5–6 weeks
    e. True

2. a. False   Appears at the age of 7–12 months
    b. False   From birth
    c. True
    d. True   And stays throughout life
    e. False   From birth

3. a. True
    b. True
    c. True   With palmar grasp
    d. False   By the age of 9 months
    e. True

4. a. True
    b. True
    c. True
    d. False
    e. True

5. a. True
    b. True
    c. False   This can be done at the age of 3 years
    d. True
    e. False   200 or more words by the age of 3 years

6. **Milestones which a normal 3-year-old child can be expected to achieve include**
   a. Catching a ball with two hands
   b. Jumping with his feet together
   c. Walking downstairs using both feet
   d. Giving their full name, address and age
   e. Lifting and replacing a cup safely

7. **Normal developmental achievement at the age of 4 years include**
   a. Climbing a ladder
   b. Walking on a narrow line backwards
   c. Naming colours
   d. Washing hands and drying them
   e. Hopping on one leg

8. **Visual development at the appropriate age includes**
   a. Neonates — watches mother during feeding
   b. 3 months — recognises small pellet on the table
   c. 12 months — picks up hundreds and thousands
   d. 2–5 years — stycar single letter recognition
   e. Over the age of 4 years — Snellen chart recognition

9. **Hearing tests at the appropriate age include**
   a. 2–3 months — loud noises, e.g. hoovering
   b. 4–7 months — sound at a distance of 15–20 cm from ear level
   c. Over the age of 7 months — distraction test
   d. 2 years — turns to voices appropriately
   e. 4 years onwards — audiometry

Answers overleaf

6. a. True   And throwing it without falling
     b. True
     c. True   And upstairs with one foot at a time
     d. False   Can give full name and age. At the age of 4 years can give name, address and age
     e. True   This can be done by the age of 2 years

7. a. True
     b. False   Only forwards
     c. True   Up to 4–5 colours
     d. True
     e. True

8. a. True
     b. False   They recognize a small pellet on the table at the age of 6 months
     c. True   Starts from the age of 10 months
     d. False   Stycar single letter test can be used from the age of 4 years onwards.
     e. False   Snellen charts can be used from the age of 7 years onwards

9. a. True
     b. False   Turns to mother's voice by this age
     c. True
     d. True   Starts at the age of 12–18 months
     e. True

10. **The development of manipulation in children is as follows**
    a. 2 years — copies circles
    b. 4 years — copies a +
    c. $3\frac{1}{2}$ years — copies bridge with building blocks
    d. 18 months — builds tower of 6 blocks
    e. 4 years — draws a man

11. **An increase in head circumference without hydrocephalus is commonly associated with**
    a. Large baby
    b. Cerebral tumour
    c. Storage disorders
    d. Neurofibromatosis
    e. Craniosynostosis

12. **The following statements relating to puberty are correct**
    a. It can be assessed accurately by chronological age
    b. In hypothalamic disease may not occur at all
    c. Disturbances in the pineal region can cause precocious puberty
    d. Lesions in the anterior part of the third ventricle can accelerate puberty
    e. Occurs earlier in African than in South American children

13. **The actions of FSH during puberty on different organs includes**
    a. Stimulating the ovarian follicles to produce oestrogen
    b. Stimulating the Leydig cells to produce testosterone
    c. Stimulating Leydig cell proliferation causing testicular enlargement
    d. A surge that causes ovulation
    e. FSH is responsible for secondary male characteristics

Answers overleaf

10. a. False   Scribbles at 2 years and draws a circle at 3 years
    b. True
    c. True   Builds a tower of three at 9–12 months, tower of six at 12 months and a tower of nine at 18–24 months
    d. True
    e. True

11. a. True   Can also be familial
    b. False
    c. True
    d. True
    e. False

12. a. False   Puberty can be assessed better by bone age
    b. True
    c. True   Which is commonest among boys
    d. False   This can delay puberty
    e. False

13. a. True
    b. False   This is the action of LH
    c. False   By seminiferous tube proliferation
    d. False   This is the action of LH
    e. False   This is the action of LH

14. The following statements relating to puberty in girls are correct
a. It begins with breast development
b. Onset is at a mean age of 11.8–12 years
c. The growth spurt occurs between stages 3 and 4 of breast development
d. Stage 3 of breast development is characterized by elevation of the areola with enlargement of breast
e. The onset of menstruation occurs at the time of the growth spurt

15. Characteristic features of true precocious puberty include
a. Activation of the hypothalamo-pituitary-gonadal axis
b. Pubertal changes are incomplete
c. Testes are greater than 2 ml in volume
d. Advanced bone age
e. Clitoromegaly

16. Common causes of true precocious puberty occurring in boys rather than girls include
a. CNS tumours
b. McCune–Albright syndrome
c. Idiopathic causes
d. Hypothyroidism
e. Neurofibromatosis

17. Causes of tall stature during childhood with final short stature include
a. Congenital adrenal hyperplasia
b. Hypothyroidism
c. Virilizing adrenal tumours
d. Hydrocephalus
e. Homocystinuria

Answers overleaf

14. a. True
b. True
c. False   Between stages 2 and 3 of breast development
d. True
e. False   It occurs after the growth spurts at stage 4 of breast development

15. a. True
b. False   Changes are complete but incomplete in pseudo-precocious puberty
c. True
d. True   Occurs in both true and pseudo-puberty
e. False   This is a feature of pseudo-precocious puberty

16. a. True   In more than 50% of boys the cause is CNS tumours but in 90% of girls it is idiopathic
b. False   Almost all those affected are girls
c. False
d. False   Both
e. False   This is not a common cause of precocious puberty in either sex

17. a. True
b. False
c. True
d. False   Normal or short stature
e. False   Tall stature

Cardiology

1. **Characteristic features of Wolff–Parkinson–White Syndrome include**
   a. An anomalous electrical connection between atria and ventricles
   b. There is earlier and slower depolarization of the ventricles resulting in a short P-R interval
   c. A short P-R interval, wide QRS, and delta wave are the main features on ECG
   d. Voltage criteria can be used in the diagnosis of ventricular hypertrophy
   e. Re-entry tachyarrhythmias are common in children

2. **In ventricular septal defects**
   a. The membranous part is typically involved
   b. The murmur radiates to the neck
   c. A mitral diastolic murmur is due to increased flow through the defect
   d. Endocarditis usually develops on the right ventricular side
   e. A significant rise in ventricular pressure is common

3. **In ventricular septal defects**
   a. Spontaneous closure occurs in more than 50% of cases in the first year of life
   b. Disappearance of the murmur in association with a loud second heart sound are signs of closure of the defect
   c. A pulmonary to systemic pressure ratio of more than 3:1 is an indication for early surgery.
   d. Exercise restriction should not apply to children with a VSD
   e. Physical growth in children with a small VSD is abnormal

4. **Characteristic features of an atrial septal defect (ASD) include**
   a. Left axis deviation with a right-bundle-branch block are the usual ECG findings with a secundum ASD
   b. Heart failure is the commonest presentation in childhood
   c. It is commonly associated with a prolonged P-R interval on ECG
   d. Eisenmenger's syndrome commonly follows an untreated ASD
   e. Atrial fibrillation usually occurs before surgical repair

Answers overleaf

1. a. True
　 b. True
　 c. True
　 d. False　As there is re-entry the voltage criteria will be affected
　 e. True

2. a. True
　 b. False
　 c. False
　 d. True
　 e. True　This is due to volume overflow

3. a. True　For small and moderate sized VSDs
　 b. False　Indicates an increase in pulmonary pressure
　 c. True
　 d. True
　 e. False　No effect on physical or mental growth of children with small VSDs

4. a. False　RBBB with right axis deviation are the commonest abnormalities in secundum ASDs
　 b. False　Heart murmur is the commonest presentation in childhood
　 c. False
　 d. False　Rare
　 e. False　Usually occurs after surgical repair

5. **The following statements relating to patent ductus arteriosus (PDA) are correct**
   a. With a PDA the pulse pressure varies with respiration
   b. Prostaglandins can be used to close a PDA
   c. Hypoxia may be the cause of the ductus arteriosus failing to close
   d. 15–20% of premature babies have a PDA
   e. Most infants with a PDA are asymptomatic

6. **Coarctation of the aorta**
   a. Is characterized by a delay in femoral pulsation
   b. May present as hypertension
   c. Is commonly associated with a bicuspid aortic valve
   d. Is the commonest cardiac lesion in Noonan's syndrome
   e. Always occurs distal to the origin of the left subclavian artery

7. **Tetralogy of Fallot is characterized by**
   a. Infundibular pulmonary stenosis
   b. Right ventricular hypertrophy
   c. A complete atrio-ventricular septal defect
   d. Pulmonary oligaemia on chest X-ray
   e. Central cyanosis appearing in the first week of life

8. **Recognized complications of untreated Fallot's tetralogy include**
   a. Cerebral abscesses
   b. Infective endocarditis
   c. Cyanotic spells
   d. Hypoglycaemia
   e. Heart failure

9. **The following statements relating to cyanotic congenital heart disease are correct**
   a. May be present without visible cyanosis in the first few days of life
   b. Fallot's tetralogy is the commonest cause
   c. Indomethacin can be used in the treatment of duct dependent defects
   d. Thrombosis is a recognized complication
   e. The oxygen dissociation curve is shifted to the right

Answers overleaf

5. a. True
   b. False   Helps to keep the duct open. Indomethacin is used to close PDAs
   c. True
   d. True
   e. True

6. a. True
   b. True   But most commonly presents as a systolic murmur or heart failure during infancy
   c. True
   d. False   Is the commonest heart lesion associated with Turner's syndrome. Noonan's is associated with pulmonary stenosis, ASD and cardiomyopathy
   e. False

7. a. True   Other features include: over-riding of the aorta, VSD and right ventricular hypertrophy
   b. True
   c. False
   d. True
   e. False

8. a. True
   b. True
   c. True
   d. False
   e. False   Rarely causes heart failure

9. a. True
   b. True
   c. False
   d. True
   e. False   **Shifted to the left**

10. Pulmonary stenosis is characterized by
  a. A loud second heart sound
  b. An ejection systolic murmur radiating to both sides of the neck
  c. Plethoric lung fields on chest X-ray
  d. Right ventricular strain on ECG
  e. A systolic thrill in the suprasternal notch

11. Surgical procedures which can be used in the treatment of transposition of the great arteries include
  a. Mustard operation
  b. Arterial switch operation
  c. Balloon septostomy
  d. Rashkind procedure
  e. Blalock Taussig shunt

12. The following statements relating to total anomalous pulmonary venous drainage are correct
  a. It may present with cyanosis in the first week of life
  b. The infra-diaphragmatic version is the commonest type
  c. Heart size is often normal on chest X-ray
  d. A systolic murmur is usually heard over the lung fields
  e. On cardiac catheterization there is a step-up in oxygen saturation from the vena cava to the right atrium

13. The following statements relating to the physiology of congestive cardiac failure are correct
  a. The end-diastolic pressures in both ventricles are increased
  b. Pulmonary artery pressure is decreased
  c. Decreased oxygen saturation in the aorta can cause pulmonary oedema
  d. Increased diastolic filling of both ventricles may cause third and fourth heart sounds
  e. Tachycardia is due to an increase in sympathetic tone

14. Drugs commonly used in the treatment of heart failure include
  a. Thiazide diuretics
  b. Digoxin
  c. Prazosin
  d. Frusemide
  e. Propranolol

Answers overleaf

10. a. True   The pulmonary component of second heart sound is loud
    b. False   The ejection systolic murmur at the left second intercostal space does not radiate to the neck
    c. False   Oligaemic lung fields on chest X-ray
    d. True   Sometimes associated with right axis deviation
    e. False   This is a characteristic feature of aortic stenosis

11. a. True
    b. True
    c. True
    d. True
    e. False   This is commonly used in Fallot's tetralogy and pulmonary atresia

12. a. True
    b. False   The cardiac and supracardiac forms are the commonest
    c. True   Especially in the infra-diaphragmatic type
    d. False   No murmurs are associated with the infradiaphragmatic type
    e. True

13. a. True   This can lead to hepatomegaly, peripheral and pulmonary oedema
    b. False
    c. False
    d. True
    e. True   Also the peripheral vascular resistance increases as the sympathetic tone increases

14. a. True
    b. True
    c. False
    d. True
    e. False

15. **Major criteria used for the diagnosis of rheumatic fever include**
  a. Arthralgia
  b. Carditis
  c. A prolonged P-R interval
  d. An increased ASO titre
  e. Erythema marginatum

16. **Organisms causing bacterial endocarditis include**
  a. Group B beta haemolytic streptococci
  b. *Haemophilus influenzae* type b
  c. *Candida albicans*
  d. Atypical bacteria
  e. *Pseudomonas aeruginosa*

17. **The following statements relating to bacterial endocarditis are true**
  a. Embolization occurs mainly as a result of immune complex phenomena
  b. Patients may be rheumatoid factor positive
  c. Serum complement levels are elevated
  d. A negative blood culture will exclude bacterial endocarditis
  e. Intravenous antibiotic therapy for 10 days is an effective treatment

18. **The following statements relating to hypertension in childhood are correct**
  a. It may present as recurrent headache
  b. 95% of cases of secondary hypertension are due to renal disease
  c. In cases of primary hyperaldosteronism it is associated with hyperkalaemia
  d. Elevated vanillmandelic acids are diagnostic of phaeochromocytoma
  e. Is defined as a diastolic blood pressure above the 95th centile on BP by age chart

Answers overleaf

15. a. False Major criteria include: carditis, arthritis, erythema marginatum chorea and subcutaneous nodules. Minor criteria include: rise in arthralgia, prolonged PR interval, fever, a high ESR and an elevated C-reactive protein

    b. True
    c. False
    d. False
    e. True

16. a. False Other bacteria include: *Staphylococcus aureus* and *Staph. albus* and alpha-haemolytic streptococcus (Viridans)

    b. False
    c. True
    d. True *Coxiella burnetii* (Q fever)
    e. False

17. a. True
    b. True
    c. False Normal or low serum complement levels
    d. False Serial blood cultures are needed for diagnosis and about 10% are blood culture negative

    e. False

18. a. True
    b. True Reflux nephropathy is the commonest cause of secondary hypertension
    c. False Hypokalaemia
    d. False Also raised in neuroblastoma
    e. True

19. Features of pericarditis include
   a. Neck pain
   b. An inverted ST wave segment on ECG
   c. Staphylococci infection is the commonest bacterial pathogen in young children
   d. Pulsus paradoxus
   e. Pulsatile liver

20. The valsava manoeuvre results in the following changes
   a. Blood pressure increases initially then falls
   b. Venous return increases
   c. Venous return is impaired with an associated tachycardia
   d. There is a rise in blood pressure with an associated bradycardia
   e. There is an increase in intrathoracic pressure

21. The following statements relating to ECGs in children are correct
   a. T wave inversion in V1, V2 and V3 is abnormal
   b. A tall R wave in V1 with a tall S wave is diagnostic of RVH in neonates
   c. A prolonged Q-T interval is found in hypercalcaemia
   d. A Q wave on the outer chest leads occurs in Duchenne muscular dystrophy
   e. The P wave is due to atrial contraction

22. Features of paroxysmal supraventricular tachycardia include
   a. It is the commonest tachyarrythmia of infants and children
   b. The incidence is approximately 1:10 000
   c. It may present with heart failure
   d. Intravenous verapamil is the treatment of choice
   e. The diving reflex can be used as first line treatment

Answers overleaf

19. a. True   Or retrosternal pain which may be relieved by sitting up
    b. False   Widespread ST segment elevation, concave upwards
    c. True
    d. True
    e. False   This is a feature of constrictive pericarditis

20. a. True
    b. False
    c. True
    d. False
    e. True

21. a. False   This is a normal variation
    b. False   Right ventricular dominance is a common ECG finding during the neonatal period
    c. False   Hypocalcaemia can cause a prolonged Q-T interval
    d. True
    e. True

22. a. True
    b. False
    c. True
    d. False   Contraindicated as it may cause bradycardia and cardiac arrest. The drug treatment of choice is adenosine
    e. True

23. **The following statments relating to syndromes associated with cardiac lesions are correct**
   a. William's syndrome — sub-valvar aortic stenosis
   b. Romano–Ward syndrome — prolonged Q-T on ECG
   c. Jervell–Lang–Niellsen syndrome — short Q-T interval
   d. Ellis–van-Creveld syndrome — atrial septal defect
   e. Holt–Oram syndrome — pulmonary stenosis

24. **The following statements regarding the action of anti-arrythmic drugs are correct**
   a. Class I drugs delay repolarization
   b. Class II drugs are calcium antagonists
   c. Class I drugs can slow the fast-rising phase of ventricular action potentials
   d. Disopyramide can be used in both atrial and ventricular arrhythmias
   e. Digoxin can shorten the refractory period in the atrioventricular node

25. **The left coronary artery supplies the left ventricle via the following branches**
   a. Anterior descending artery
   b. Posterior descending artery
   c. Circumflex artery
   d. Acute marginal branch
   e. Intermediate branch of the left coronary artery

Answers overleaf

23. a. False Supravalvar aortic stenosis, hypercalcaemia and elfin facies
    b. True
    c. False Prolonged Q-T interval and deafness
    d. True   Postaxial polydactyly
    e. False ASD and radial aplasia

24. a. False
    b. False
    c. True
    d. True
    e. False

25. a. True
    b. False This is a branch of the right coronary artery
    c. True
    d. False This is a branch of the right coronary artery
    e. True

Respiratory

1. **The following statements relating to cystic fibrosis are correct**
   a. The commonest mutation results in the loss of phenylalanine at position 508
   b. The gene is located on chromosome 7
   c. The carrier rate is 1 in 40
   d. Intrauterine diagnosis is not possible
   e. Fertility is normal in females

2. **Substances which can cause asthma include**
   a. Aspirin
   b. Paracetamol
   c. Silicone
   d. Isocynates
   e. Cotton dust

3. **Factors causing a shift of the oxyhaemoglobin dissociation curve to the right include**
   a. Increased temperature
   b. A low $P_a\text{CO}_2$
   c. A low 2,3 DPG level
   d. Alkalosis
   e. Anaemia

4. **Wheezing can be associated with the following conditions**
   a. Respiratory syncitial virus infection
   b. Left ventricular failure
   c. Bronchiectasis
   d. Extrinsic allergic alveolitis
   e. Cow's milk protein intolerance

5. **The following drugs may cause pulmonary fibrosis**
   a. Aspirin
   b. Busulphan
   c. Bleomycin
   d. Erythromycin
   e. Nitrofurantoin

Answers overleaf

1. a. True
   b. True   Delta F508 occurs in 80% of the affected
                 population. The gene is located on chromosome
                 ~~X~~7
   c. False   It is approximately 1 in 20
   d. False
   e. ~~True~~   Males are infertile
        false   low in Females.

2. a. True
   b. False
   c. False
   d. True
   e. True

3. a. True   The oxygen dissociation curve is shifted to the
                 right by acidosis, hypoxia, anaemia, an increase in
                 2,3 DPG levels, high temperature and high
                 altitude
   b. False   Shifted to the left by alkalosis, low temperature
                 and a decrease in 2,3 DPG levels
   c. False
   d. False
   e. True

4. a. True   Inhalation of foreign bodies, cystic fibrosis and
                 aspiration may cause wheeze
   b. True
   c. True
   d. False   Characterized by late inspiratory crepitations with
                 no wheeze
   e. True

5. a. False
   b. True
   c. True
   d. False
   e. True

6. **Pleural effusions are associated with the following conditions**
   a. Post-cardiac surgery
   b. Pneumonia
   c. Cardiac failure
   d. Lung abscesses
   e. Cystic fibrosis

7. **In normal lungs**
   a. The right lung is higher than the left one
   b. The lingula is part of the left lower lobe
   c. All bronchi and bronchioles have cartilage in their walls
   d. The lymphatic drainage of the left lung is via the left subclavian vein
   e. The visceral pleura is supplied by the phrenic nerve

8. **Characteristic features of a respiratory acidosis include**
   a. A fall in blood pH
   b. An increase in $P_a\text{co}_2$
   c. A decrease in $P_a\text{co}_2$
   d. Decreased renal bicarbonate excretion
   e. An increased affinity of haemoglobin for oxygen

9. **The following are features of type I respiratory failure**
   a. A high $P_a\text{co}_2$
   b. A normal $P_a\text{o}_2$
   c. Cystic fibrosis is a possible cause
   d. Hypoventilation is an aetiological factor
   e. It may result from depression of the respiratory centre by drugs

10. **In alveolar capillary block**
   a. Vital capacity is high
   b. Forced expiratory volume is normal
   c. PEFR is low
   d. Diffusion capacity is normal
   e. Collagen disorders are a possible cause

Answers overleaf

6. a. True
   b. True
   c. True
   d. True
   e. False   Transudative pleural effusions are associated with heart failure, renal failure, JCA and ascites. Exudative pleural effusions are associated with malignancy and lung infection

7. a. True
   b. False   The Lingula is a part of left upper lobe
   c. False   Bronchi have cartilage but not bronchioles
   d. True   Whilst that of the right lung is via the thoracic duct to SVC
   e. False

8. a. True
   b. True
   c. False
   d. False   Renal bicarbonate excretion is increased
   e. False   The affinity of haemoglobin for oxygen is decreased

9. a. True   Low P_aO_2 and a high or normal P_aCO_2
   b. False
   c. True
   d. True
   e. True

10. a. False   Alveolar-capillary block occurs in restrictive lung diseases
    b. True
    c. False
    d. False
    e. True

11. Lung function in restrictive lung disease is characterized by
   a. A reduction in FEV_1
   b. A normal diffusion capacity
   c. A low FEV_1/FVC ratio
   d. A low P_aCO_2
   e. A reduction in total lung capacity

12. Miliary tuberculosis is characterized by
   a. Few chest signs
   b. Splenomegaly
   c. Low temperature
   d. CSF with a high protein high level
   e. A diagnostic appearance on chest X-ray

13. In the treatment of asthma
   a. A large volume spacer device can be used by most toddlers
   b. A metered dose inhaler is usually used by children over the age of 3 years
   c. Sodium chromoglycate is the first line prophylactic treatment in children
   d. Slow release aminophylline may be used in children
   e. Inhaled steroids are likely to affect the growth of children at a dose 400–800 μg daily

14. Acute onset of stridor may be due to
   a. A vascular ring
   b. Bacterial tracheitis
   c. A foreign body
   d. Laryngomalacia
   e. Tonsillitis

15. A low P_aO_2 with low P_aCO_2 may be associated with
   a. Asthma
   b. Left ventricular failure
   c. Hysteria
   d. Cystic fibrosis
   e. Kyphoscoliosis

Answers overleaf

11. a. True
    b. False   Diffusion capacity is low
    c. False FEV_1/FVC is high or normal. Low in obstructive lung disease
    d. True
    e. True

12. a. True
    b. True
    c. False
    d. True   And a low sugar with a high lymphocyte count
    e. False   Miliary shadows are seen in other infections

13. a. True
    b. False
    c. True
    d. True
    e. False   Usually no clinically discernible effect on growth at that dose

14. a. False   Chronic
    b. True   Also epiglottitis and laryngeotracheobronchitis
    c. True
    d. False   Chronic
    e. True

15. a. True   Hypocapnia occurs before hypercapnia
    b. True
    c. True   Hyperventilation is associated with a low P_aCO_2
    d. False
    e. False   Hypercapnia and hypoxia

16. Miliary calcification of the lungs may be due to
    a. Tuberculosis
    b. Measles
    c. Chickenpox
    d. Histoplasmosis
    e. HIV

17. Bronchiectasis may be associated with
    a. Mumps
    b. Chickenpox
    c. Dextrocardia
    d. Foreign body inhalation
    e. Allergic bronchopulmonary aspergillosis

18. In respiratory alkalosis
    a. Blood pH is increased
    b. P_aO_2 is increased
    c. Hyperventilation is a common cause
    d. Serum bicarbonate levels are increased
    e. Cerebral blood flow is increased

Answers overleaf

16. a. True
    b. False
    c. True
    d. True
    e. True

17. a. False
    b. False
    c. True   As well as measles and cystic fibrosis
    d. True
    e. True

18. a. True
    b. False P_aO_2 is normal
    c. True
    d. False
    e. False

Gastroenterology

1. **The following statements relating to gastric acid secretion are correct**
   a. Gastric acid secretion is controlled mainly by the vagus nerve
   b. 70% of children with duodenal ulcers have normal gastric acid secretion
   c. It is reduced by suppression of gastrin secretion
   d. Enteroglucagon increases acid secretion
   e. It is secreted by the chief cells in the gastric mucosa

2. **True or false**
   a. Gastrin is secreted by parietal cells on the greater curvature of the stomach
   b. Gastrin output increases in response to high pH of the stomach contents
   c. Gastrin acts directly on digested protein
   d. Parietal cells have receptors for acetylcholine
   e. Gastric emptying will be slowed by a low pH

3. **True or false**
   a. Cholecystokinin production is stimulated by the presence of protein in the duodenum
   b. Secretin acts directly in the lumen of the duodenum
   c. Pancreatic enzyme secretion is stimulated by cholecystokinin
   d. Secretin stimulates production of bicarbonate by the duodenum
   e. Cholecystokinin causes gall bladder contraction

4. **Absorption of carbohydrates is characterized by**
   a. 60% of dietary carbohydrates are in the form of starch
   b. Lactose is digested to produce glucose
   c. Glucose and galactose are actively transported across the cell membranes
   d. Fructose is transported passively across cell membranes
   e. Glucose will be absorbed following gastroenteritis

Answers overleaf

1. a. True
   b. True
   c. True   Suppression of gastrin secretion can be due to a low antral PH, glucagon and secretin. Fat in the duodenum induces secretion of enteroglucagon, GIP and neurotensin, which inhibit gastrin secretion. Other inhibitory factors include: vagotomy, atropine, insulin, VIP, H_2 antagonists, anticholinergic agents and acid pump inhibitors (omeprazole)
   d. False
   e. False

2. a. False   By parietal cells in the antral mucosa
   b. True   And ingestion of protein
   c. False
   d. True   And glucagon
   e. True   As well as secretin and enteroglucagon hormones

3. a. True   And fats
   b. False   It is secreted by the duodenal mucosa to stimulate pancreatic bicarbonate secretion
   c. True
   d. False
   e. True

4. a. True   Starch is broken down by amylase
   b. True   And sucrose hydrolysed to glucose
   c. True
   d. True   Facilitated diffusion
   e. False   Fructose is well absorbed after gastroenteritis but not glucose or galactose

5. Physiological changes occurring in pyloric stenosis include
   a. An elevated serum urea
   b. A metabolic acidosis
   c. Hypocalcaemia
   d. Hyperchloraemia
   e. Hypokalaemia

6. True or false
   a. Hypocalcaemia can cause constipation
   b. A flat brush border on jejunal biopsy is diagnostic of coeliac disease
   c. Appetite is good in children with coeliac disease
   d. Meconium ileus equivalent causes constipation
   e. Lead poisoning can cause diarrhoea

7. The following statements relating to coeliac disease are correct
   a. There is subtotal villous atrophy on microscopy
   b. An increase in antigliaden antibodies is diagnostic
   c. Patients should be re-biopsied on a gluten-free diet
   d. There is an increased incidence of lymphoma
   e. It is associated with acrodermatitis enteropathica

8. Crohn's disease is characterized by the following features
   a. It is more common in boys
   b. It can present with anaemia
   c. It involves the colon in 40% of cases
   d. The terminal ileum is commonly involved
   e. Aphthous ulcers are pathognomonic

9. Features suggestive of Crohn's disease rather than ulcerative colitis include
   a. Crypt abscesses
   b. Non-granulomatous caseating lesions
   c. Lead-pipe appearance on barium enema
   d. Shortening of the intestine
   e. Transmural inflammation

Answers overleaf

5. a. True
   b. False
   c. False
   d. False
   e. True

6. a. False   Hypercalcaemia
   b. False   Flat jejunal biopsy can be seen in coeliac disease, postenteritis syndrome, cow's milk protein intolerance, giardiasis, protein energy malnutrition, hypogammaglobulinaemia and tropical sprue
   c. False   They are anorexic
   d. True
   e. False   Chronic lead poisoning causes constipation

7. a. True
   b. False   Present but not diagnostic. It is a useful screening test
   c. True
   d. True   Mainly intestinal lymphoma
   e. False

8. a. False   Equal in both sexes
   b. True   Other features include: loss of weight, short stature, abdominal pain, arthritis, pyoderma gangrenosum, diarrhoea, anal fissure and anorexia
   c. False   Isolated colon involvement can occur in 20%
   d. True   Crohn's disease affects the gastrointestinal tract from mouth to anus
   e. False

9. a. False
   b. True   Their presence should always suggest Crohn's disease.
   c. False   This is the appearance of ulcerative colitis on X-ray
   d. False
   e. True

10. The following statements relating to Hirschsprung's disease are correct
  a. There is an absence of adrenergic sympathetic nerve endings in the ganglion cells (Auerbach's and Meissner's plexus) in the distal segment of the gut
  b. It is more common in females than males
  c. Delayed passage of meconium is an early presentation
  d. It may present with alternating periods of diarrhoea and constipation
  e. Older children have abdominal distension

11. In the liver
  a. Hepatic lobules are composed of efferent vein, hepatocytes and sinusoids
  b. Portal tracts contain the hepatic artery, hepatic vein, bile ductules and supporting structures
  c. Sinusoids contain endothelial, Kupffer and Ito cells
  d. Bile ducts and hepatocytes are derived from mesoderm
  e. During intrauterine life the umbilical venous blood is diverted to the SVC via the ductus venosus and portal vein

12. The liver may be involved in
  a. Galactosaemia
  b. AIDS
  c. Coeliac disease
  d. Cystic fibrosis
  e. Leptospirosis

13. Reye's syndrome
  a. Is characterized by encephalopathy and disturbance of liver function
  b. May follow a viral illness
  c. A high serum bilirubin is a common finding
  d. A serum aminotransaminase up to 100 times greater than normal is often found
  e. Vomiting may be the earliest symptom

Answers overleaf

10. a. True
   b. True
   c. True
   d. True
   e. True   With faecal soiling

11. a. True
   b. False   Portal tract components include: hepatic artery, portal vein, bile ductules and supporting structures
   c. True
   d. False   Kupffer cells, endothelial cells, bile ducts and hepatocytes are derived from endoderm
   e. False   Deviated to IVC

12. a. True
   b. True   Liver abscess or Kaposi's sarcoma
   c. True   Fatty infiltration
   d. True   Liver cirrhosis
   e. True   Hepatitis

13. a. True   Fatty infiltration and mitochondrial changes are the main changes in the liver
   b. True   Chickenpox is the commonest. Salicylate ingestion is a risk factor and should be avoided in viral illnesses in children under the age of 12 years.
   c. False   Serum bilirubin is normal, ammonia is high and blood sugar is low
   d. True
   e. True   Which is profuse and persistent

14. **The following laboratory results are compatible with a diagnosis of chronic active hepatitis**
    a. ANF is positive in 80% of patients
    b. Mitochondrial antibodies are found in > 90% of patients
    c. Elevated serum immunoglobulin levels
    d. Low alpha-globulin levels
    e. High alkaline phosphatase levels

15. **In Wilson's disease**
    a. The inheritance is autosomal recessive
    b. There is a defect in copper metabolism
    c. Neurological problems are found more commonly in children than adults
    d. There are no benefits from starting D-penicillinamine treatment early
    e. A Kaiser-Fleisher ring is pathognomonic

16. **Causes of intrahepatic portal hypertension in infants and children include**
    a. The Budd-Chiari syndrome
    b. Hepatic vein thrombosis
    c. Multiple granulomata
    d. Portal vein thrombosis
    e. Veno-occlusive disease of the liver

17. **The following statements relating to ascites are correct**
    a. Transudative ascites has a low protein concentration
    b. Exudative ascites can be due to malignancy
    c. It may predispose to haemorrhage if cirrhosis is the cause
    d. Hypokalaemia is a commonly associated electrolytic disturbance
    e. Hypertonic saline is not used in the treatment

Answers overleaf

14. a. False ANF is found in 50% of patients with CAH
    b. False Smooth muscle antibodies is found in 65% of patients with CAH
    c. True
    d. False Are high
    e. True   Aminotransferases (AST), bilirubin, gammaglutamyltransferase are elevated. Albumin is low

15. a. True
    b. True   The disturbance of copper metabolism is characterized by a decreased serum concentration of the copper-carrying protein [caeruloplasmin], and by a failure of copper to be incorporated with caeruloplasmin
    c. False Wilson's disease in children commonly presents with liver disease as an early manifestation
    d. False There is a dramatic improvement in neurological symptoms, but the hepatic and psychiatric symptoms are less predictable
    e. True

16. a. True   Hepatic causes include: Budd-Chiari syndrome, cardiac disease and IVC web.
              Pre-hepatic: portal vein thrombosis, arterio-venous fistulae and chronic pancreatitis. Intrahepatic: cirrhosis
    b. True   This is the cause of Budd-Chiari syndrome
    c. True
    d. False
    e. True

17. a. True   Causes include heart failure and nephrotic syndrome
    b. True   And infection, intestinal obstruction
    c. True
    d. True   And hyponatraemia
    e. True

18. Biliary cirrhosis may be due to
   a. Ulcerative colitis
   b. Veno-occlusive disease
   c. Gaucher's disease
   d. Extra hepatic biliary atresia
   e. Cystic fibrosis

19. Known causes of pancreatitis include
   a. Polyarteritis nodosa
   b. Paracetamol poisoning
   c. Trauma
   d. Hypercalcaemia
   e. Rubella infection

20. Features more common in Crohn's disease than ulcerative colitis include
   a. Abdominal pain
   b. Bloody diarrhoea
   c. Pyoderma gangrenosum
   d. Arthritis
   e. Perianal lesions

Answers overleaf

18. a. True   And Crohn's disease
     b. False   This can cause post-hepatic cirrhosis
     c. False   Causes hepatomegaly without splenomegaly
     d. True
     e. True

19. a. True
     b. False
     c. True
     d. True
     e. True

20. a. True
     b. False   More common in ulcerative colitis
     c. False
     d. False   Occurs in both conditions
     e. True

Metabolic disorders

1. **The following statements relating to insulin-dependent diabetes mellitus are correct**
   a. A glucose tolerance test is required for diagnosis in all children
   b. 10–30% may present with diabetic ketoacidosis (DKA)
   c. A fasting venous blood sugar of > 10 mmol/l 2 hours after a 75-g glucose load is diagnostic of diabetes mellitus
   d. Microalbuminuria has no long-term sequelae
   e. A glycolysated haemoglobin of 10% is an indication of good control

2. **Characteristic features of the Wolfram syndrome include**
   a. Autosomal dominant inheritance
   b. Deafness
   c. Short stature
   d. Progressive optic atrophy
   e. Half of affected children develop diabetes insipidus in the second decade

3. **Insulin**
   a. Is a C-peptide hormone secreted by the B-cells of the pancreas
   b. Is antagonized by growth hormone
   c. Human purified insulin has significant antigenic side-effects
   d. Can increase lipolysis
   e. May decrease glycogenolysis

4. **Syndromes associated with an impaired glucose tolerance include**
   a. Ataxic telangiectasia
   b. Friedreich's ataxia
   c. Refsum's syndrome
   d. Down's syndrome
   e. Turner's syndrome

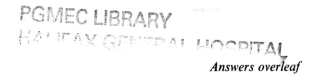

Answers overleaf

75

1. a. False Rarely required in children if a random blood
                sugar level is high
   b. True
   c. True
   d. False Predictive of a 10% risk of developing
                nephropathy in the next 10 years
   e. False This is an indication of poor control

2. a. True   Diabetes mellitus, diabetes insipidus, deafness and
                optic atrophy are the characteristic features of
                Wolfram's syndrome
   b. True
   c. False
   d. True
   e. False A third of them develop diabetes insipidus by the
                2nd decade of life

3. a. True
   b. True   And glucagon
   c. False The bovine and pig insulins have most antigenic
                side-effects
   d. True   And gluconeogenesis
   e. False Insulin increases glycogenolysis and proteolysis

4. a. True   Duchenne muscular dystrophy, cystic fibrosis,
                Cushing's syndrome and Prader Willi syndrome
                can all be associated with glucose intolerance
   b. True
   c. False
   d. True
   e. True

5. Recognized complication of insulin-dependent diabetes mellitus include
   a. Necrobiosis diabeticorum lipoidica
   b. Moniliasis
   c. Delayed puberty
   d. Retinopathy
   e. Erythema annulare

6. Hyperinsulinaemia can be associated with
   a. Erythroblastosis
   b. Fructosaemia
   c. Nesidioblastosis
   d. Maple syrup urine disease
   e. Proprionic acidaemia

7. Ketoacidosis is known to be due to
   a. Maple syrup urine disease
   b. McArdle's disease (type V glycogen storage disease)
   c. Organic acidaemia
   d. Von Gierke's disease (type I glycogen storage disease)
   e. Homocystinuria

8. Hyperammonaemia and hypoglycaemia can be associated with the following conditions
   a. Urea cycle defects (e.g. ornithine transcarboxylase deficiency)
   b. Methylmalonaemic acidaemia
   c. Hunter's syndrome
   d. Von Gierke's disease (type Ib)
   e. Reye's syndrome

9. Characteristic features of galactosaemia include
   a. Onset is usually in the first month of life
   b. Vomiting is progressive
   c. Late cataract formation
   d. Tolerance of cow's milk better than human milk
   e. IQ may be low even with early treatment

Answers overleaf

5. a. True   May be the earliest manifestation of DM
   b. True   Vaginal moniliasis is the commonest
   c. True   Growth also delayed if DM is not well controlled
   d. True   Is common after the first 15 years of DM
   e. True

6. a. True   In infants of diabetic mothers
   b. False
   c. True
   d. False
   e. False

7. a. True
   b. False   McArdle's disease characterised by muscle pain after exercise
   c. True
   d. True
   e. False

8. a. True   They usually die early
   b. True
   c. False   This is one of the mucopolysaccharridoses
   d. False
   e. True

9. a. True   It usually presents early with jaundice, hepatomegaly, vomiting, hypoglycaemia, poor feeding and poor weight gain
   b. True
   c. False   Cataract and aminoaciduria may be an early manifestation
   d. False
   e. True

10. Features of the mucopolysaccharidoses include
   a. Type I (Hurler's) — dysostosis multiplex
   b. Type III (Sanfilippo's) — normal intelligence
   c. Type IV (Marquio's) — elevated urinary keratan sulphate excretion
   d. Type VI (Maroteaux-Lamy) — hepatosplenomegaly
   e. Type II (Hunter's) — cloudy cornea

11. A cherry red macula can be associated with
   a. Gaucher's disease
   b. Generalized gangliosidoses
   c. Niemann-Pick's disease type A and C
   d. Batten's disease
   e. Tay-Sach's disease

12. Features of Type IIa hyperlipidaemia include
   a. High cholesterol with low triglyceride levels
   b. A cholesterol level in homozygous individuals of 7–10 mmol/l
   c. Retinitis pigmentosa as a late consequence
   d. Turbid serum
   e. Xanthomata

Answers overleaf

10. a. True
    b. False   Mental retardation is a common feature
    c. True   Normal intelligence, skeletal deformity and increase urinary keratan sulphate excretion are characteristic features of type IV
    d. True   Stiff joints and elevated urinary dermatan sulphate
    e. False

11. a. False
    b. True
    c. True   Niemann-Pick's disease is due to sphingomyelinase deficiency which leads to accumulation of sphingomyelin and cholesterol in effected tissues
    d. False
    e. True

12. a. False   Both are high
    b. False   Heterozygotes have a level of 20 mmol/l and homozygous individuals 25 mmol/l
    c. False   A common feature of abetalipoproteinaemia
    d. False   Occurs in type I
    e. True

Endocrinology

1. **The following statements relating to the hypothalamus are correct**
   a. The neurosecretory cells are osmoreceptors
   b. Oxytocin and vasopressin are the only neurohumoral substances
   c. Vasopressin is usually secreted by the hypothalamus
   d. Oxytocin stimulates milk release
   e. Vasopressin pressor effects are produced by physiological rather than pharmacological quantities of the hormone

2. **With regards to calcitonin**
   a. Its function is dependent on parathyroid hormone
   b. High doses can increase the urinary excretion of parathyroid hormone
   c. Its secretion is regulated by plasma calcium levels
   d. It is secreted by the chief cells of the parathyroid gland
   e. It inhibits PTH-induced bone resorption

3. **Causes of polyuria and polydipsia include**
   a. Hypokalaemia
   b. Hypercalcaemia
   c. Urinary tract infection
   d. Chronic renal failure
   e. Nephrogenic diabetes insipidus

4. **Causes of SIADH (inappropriate anti-diuretic hormone secretion) include**
   a. Pneumonia
   b. Guillain-Barre syndrome
   c. Head injury
   d. Vincristine
   e. Status asthmaticus

5. **Laboratory findings in SIADH include**
   a. A high urine osmolality
   b. A high blood osmolality
   c. Hypokalaemia
   d. Hyponatraemia
   e. A high blood urea

Answers overleaf

1. a. True   And volume receptors
   b. False   Others are neurophysin I and II
   c. False
   d. True
   e. False   Pharmacological quantities of vasopressin have a pressor effect

2. a. False   Calcitonin function is independent of parathyroid hormone
   b. True
   c. True
   d. False   Calcitonin is secreted by the parafollicular cells of the thyroid gland
   e. True

3. a. False
   b. True
   c. False
   d. True
   e. True

4. a. True
   b. True
   c. True
   d. True
   e. True

5. a. True
   b. False
   c. False
   d. True   Serum chloride is low and serum bicarbonate is normal
   e. False

6. **The following statements relating to parathyroid hormone function are correct**
   a. It inhibits phosphate reabsorption by the renal tubules
   b. It reduces calcium levels in extracellular fluid
   c. It stimulates calcium resorption from bone in the presence of 1,25-dihydroxycholecalciferol
   d. It decreases calcium reabsorption by the renal tubules
   e. It inhibits acidification of the urine

7. **The following statements relating to the pituitary gland are correct**
   a. The anterior lobe includes the pars tuberalis, pars distalis, pars intermedia and pars nervosa
   b. It lies within the dura mater
   c. There is a subarachnoid space within the sella
   d. The optic chiasm lies anteriorly to the gland
   e. It is derived from the endoderm of the buccal cavity known as Rathke's pouch

8. **In hyperpituitarism (gigantism)**
   a. Basophilic adenoma is the commonest cause
   b. Rapid linear growth is a common finding
   c. There is an increased susceptibility to infection
   d. Hyperglycaemia is rare
   e. Suppression of plasma growth hormone in response to oral glucose is a diagnostic test

9. **Craniopharyngiomas**
   a. Are derived from the remnants of Rathke's pouch
   b. Account for 5–15% of intracranial tumours in children
   c. Invariably cause short stature
   d. An upper quadrantic hemianopia is a common feature
   e. Obesity occurs in only 20% of cases

Answers overleaf

6. a. True
    b. False   Increases both the plasma and extracellular calcium levels
    c. True
    d. False   Increases calcium reabsorption by the renal tubules
    e. True

7. a. False   Except the pars nervosa
    b. True
    c. False
    d. True
    e. True

8. a. False   Eosinophilic
    b. True
    c. True
    d. False   Common (10% of cases)
    e. False

9. a. True
    b. True
    b. True
    d. False   Bitemporal visual field defects
    e. False   In 50% of patients

10. **The following statements relating to the adrenal gland are correct**
    a. The three layers of the adrenal cortex from outside to inside are the zona glomerulosa, zona fasiculata and zona reticularis
    b. Aldosterone is synthesized by the zona reticularis
    c. Glucocorticosteroids are synthesized by the zona glomerulosa
    d. Glucocorticosteroid precursors are stored in the zona fasiculata
    e. Androgens are produced by the zona reticularis

11. **Hyperaldosteronism with high plasma renin levels can be found in**
    a. Pyloric stenosis
    b. Pseudohypoaldosteronism
    c. Primary hyperaldosteronism
    d. Cystic fibrosis
    e. Bartter's syndrome

12. **Recognized features of pseudohypoparathyroidism include**
    a. A low serum parathyroid hormone level
    b. A low serum calcium with a high serum phosphate
    c. Short third and fourth metacarpals
    d. Intracranial calcification
    e. Mental retardation

13. **Actions of the catecholamines include**
    a. Adrenaline increases diastolic blood pressure
    b. Noradrenaline slows the heart rate in the isolated heart
    c. Peripheral vascular resistance is increased by adrenaline
    d. Adrenaline relaxes the smooth muscle of the intestinal sphincters
    e. Adrenaline inhibits hepatic glycogenolysis

Answers overleaf

10. a. True
    b. False   By the zona glomerulosa
    c. False   By the zona reticularis
    d. True
    e. True   And by the zona fasiculata

11. a. True
    b. False   Low serum renin level
    c. False   Low serum renin level
    d. True
    e. True

12. a. False
    b. True
    c. True
    d. True
    e. True

13. a. False   Noradrenaline increases both systolic and diastolic while adrenaline increases only systolic blood pressure
    b. True   Adrenaline increases heart rate and cardiac output
    c. False   Coronary blood flow and peripheral vascular resistance are decreased by adrenaline and increased by noradrenaline
    d. True
    e. False   It stimulates glycogenolysis

14. True or false
   a. The development of the female genitalia is hormone dependent
   b. Testosterone acts locally to stimulate the development of the Wolffian duct to form the internal male genitalia
   c. Development of the external and internal genitalia in females is stimulated by androgens
   d. Female pseudohermaphrodites have palpable gonads
   e. The commonest cause of female pseudohermaphroditism is congenital adrenal hyperplasia

15. The testicular feminization syndrome is characterized by
   a. A karyotype of 46 XY
   b. Incomplete androgen insensitivity
   c. Normal breast development at puberty
   d. Normal internal female genitalia
   e. An X-linked inheritance

16. Causes of goitrous hypothyroidism include
   a. Autoimmune thyroiditis
   b. Pituitary tumours
   c. Pendred's syndrome
   d. Iodine deficiency
   e. Sulphonamides

17. Diagnostic tests for hypothyroidism include
   a. X-ray of the femoral epiphysis
   b. A raised serum TSH
   c. A low total serum T4
   d. A high serum T3(resin) uptake
   e. An increased free T4 index

Answers overleaf

14. a. False
b. True
c. True
d. False
e. True

15. a. True
b. False   Complete insensitivity
c. True
d. False   There are only rudimentary internal female
genitalia
e. True

16. a. True
b. False
c. True
d. True
e. True

17. a. False
b. True
c. True
d. False
e. False

Haematology

1. **In normal bone marrow**
   a. Normoblasts are the precursors of red cells
   b. The cytoplasm changes from red to blue as the red cells become more mature
   c. Myeloblasts have a high cytoplasm to nuclear ratio
   d. Lymphoblasts are more prominent in infant bone marrow
   e. Megakaryocytes have a single large nucleus

2. **Microcytic red cells are commonly seen in**
   a. Sideroblastic anaemia
   b. Chronic heavy metal poisoning
   c. Thalassaemia intermedia
   d. Liver disease
   e. Chronic renal failure

3. **Macrocytic red cells are found in the following conditions**
   a. Folate deficiency
   b. Aplastic anaemia
   c. The Blackfan–Diamond syndrome
   d. Splenic pooling
   e. Chronic blood loss

4. **Target cells are seen on blood films in the following conditions**
   a. Sickle cell anaemia
   b. Liver disease
   c. Lead poisoning
   d. Post-splenectomy
   e. Haemolytic-uraemic syndrome

5. **The following red cell morphology on blood film is associated with**
   a. Polychromasia — haemolytic anaemia
   b. Spherocytes — acute blood loss
   c. Howell-Jolly bodies — hypersplenism
   d. Acanthocytes — abetalipoproteinaemia
   e. Heinz bodies — spherocytosis

Answers overleaf

1. a. True
   b. True
   c. False   Myeloblasts have a high nuclear to cytoplasmic ratio
   d. True
   e. False   Multinucleated

2. a. True   And iron deficiency anaemia
   b. True
   c. True   Thalassaemia trait, intermedia and major all cause microcytic appearances on blood film
   d. False
   e. False

3. a. True   Also seen in Vitamin B_{12} deficiency and liver disease
   b. False   Normoblastic
   c. False   Normoblasts on bone marrow biopsy
   d. False   Normocytic
   e. False   Normoblastic and/or microcytic red blood cells

4. a. True   Target cells can be seen on blood films in both iron deficiency and the haemoglobinopathies
   b. True
   c. False   Punctate basophilia is a characteristic finding in lead poisoning
   d. True
   e. False   Burr cells are commonly associated with haemolytic uraemic syndrome

5. a. True
   b. False   Seen in hereditary spherocytosis and autoimmune haemolytic anaemias
   c. False   Howell-Jolly bodies are seen post-splenectomy and in hyposplenism
   d. True   And liver disease
   e. False   Found in glucose-6-phosphate dehydrogenase deficiency

6. In iron deficiency anaemia
 a. Serum iron levels are low
 b. The red cell count is normal
 c. MCH is reduced
 d. HbA_2 is increased
 e. Total iron binding capacity is normal

7. Characteristic features of sideroblastic anaemia include
 a. X-linked recessive inheritance
 b. Normocytic hypochromic anaemia
 c. An elevated serum iron
 d. It may be due to isoniazid treatment
 e. Normal cells on bone marrow examination

8. In immune haemolytic anaemia
 a. Cold antibodies (IgM) may be secondary to EBV infection
 b. A positive indirect Coomb's test is diagnostic
 c. Haemoglobinuria is common
 d. IgG antibody immune haemolytic anaemia (IHA) has a good prognosis
 e. There may be a response to steroid therapy

9. Drugs which can cause haemolysis in glucose-6-phosphate dehydrogenase deficiency include
 a. Phenytoin
 b. Primaquine
 c. Nitrofurantoin
 d. Salicylates
 e. Chloramphenicol

10. In Henoch-Schonlein purpura
 a. Bleeding time is prolonged
 b. There is a vasculitis
 c. Nephritis occurs in about 10% of cases
 d. There is a good response to treatment with steroids
 e. Blood pressure is often raised

Answers overleaf

6. a. True
   b. False
   c. True   MCV is also low
   d. False
   e. False

7. a. True
   b. True
   c. True
   d. True
   e. False   Ring sideroblasts on bone marrow

8. a. True   And mycoplasma pneumonia
   b. False   Direct Coombs' test is positive
   c. True
   d. False
   e. True

9. a. False
   b. True
   c. True
   d. True
   e. True

10. a. False
    b. True
    c. True   Other complications include intussusception
    d. False
    e. False

11. In haemophilia
   a. Inheritance is X-linked dominant
   b. The partial thromboplastin time (PTT) is prolonged
   c. The bleeding time is prolonged
   d. The prothrombin time is prolonged
   e. Female carriers can show signs of the disease

12. In disseminated intravascular coagulation (DIC)
   a. The bleeding time is prolonged
   b. Septicaemia is the commonest cause in babies
   c. Burr cells are found on the peripheral blood film
   d. Fibrin degradation products are low
   e. Fresh frozen plasma is not an effective treatment

13. A prolonged prothrombin time is associated with the following conditions
   a. Liver disease
   b. Factor VIII, XII and XI deficiency
   c. Vitamin K deficiency
   d. Warfarin therapy
   e. Henoch–Schonlein purpura

14. Features of thalassaemia include
   a. Autosomal dominant inheritance
   b. Excess production of a globin chain
   c. Increased HbF
   d. Increased TIBC
   e. The gene is located on chromosome 11

15. Recognized causes of a lymphocytosis include
   a. Brucellosis
   b. Infectious mononucleosis
   c. Tuberculosis
   d. Diabetes mellitus
   e. Still's disease

Answers overleaf

11. a. False   X-linked recessive
    b. True
    c. False   Normal
    d. False   Normal
    e. True

12. a. True
    b. True
    c. True
    d. False
    e. False   Fresh frozen plasma or cryoprecipitate are used to replace the missing coagulation factors

13. a. True
    b. False   This is a cause of prolonged PTT
    c. True
    d. True
    e. False

14. a. True
    b. False   Defective production of alpha- or beta-globin chain
    c. True   And HbA$_2$
    d. False
    e. True

15. a. True
    b. True
    c. True
    d. False
    e. True

16. Microangiopathic haemolytic anaemia is associated with
a. The haemolytic uraemic syndrome
b. Acute myeloblastic leukaemia
c. Disseminated malignancy
d. Septicaemia
e. Strawberry naevae

17. Splenectomy is a useful therapeutic procedure in
a. Leukaemia
b. β thalassaemia major
c. Elliptocytosis
d. Acute idiopathic thrombocytopenic purpura
e. Hereditary spherocytosis

18. The following statements relating to polycythemia rubra vera are correct
a. The ESR is raised
b. There is a shift of the dissociation oxygen curve to the right
c. There is an increased incidence of gout
d. Lymphocyte alkaline phosphatase levels are low
e. Bleeding may occur

19. Poor prognostic features in acute lymphoblastic leukaemia (ALL) include
a. Age < 1 year or > 10 years old at diagnosis
b. A mediastinal mass
c. Males
d. WBCs > 20 000 at presentation
e. B-cell type

20. The tumour lysis syndrome is characterized by
a. Hyperkalaemia
b. Hypocalcaemia
c. Hyperphosphataemia
d. Its prevention may be possible by giving allopurinol before induction
e. The blood pH is high

Answers overleaf

16. a. True
b. True
c. True
d. True
e. False

17. a. False
b. True
c. True
d. False May be applied to chronic ITP
e. True

18. a. False Low or normal
b. True
c. True Due to high level of urates
d. False Normal or high neutrophil alkaline phosphatase level
e. True As well as peptic ulceration

19. a. True
b. True
c. True
d. ~~True~~ False.
e. ~~False~~ True

20. a. True
b. ~~True~~ False.
c. True
d. True High fluid intake fluid and allopurinol
e. False

21. Features of Hodgkin's lymphoma in children include
a. Pruritis
b. Night sweats
c. Superior vena cava obstruction syndrome
d. Proteinuria
e. Jaundice

22. Poor prognostic indicators in Hodgkin's lymphoma include
a. A high ESR
b. Fever
c. A low lymphocyte count
d. Mediastinal mass
e. Anaemia

23. In Burkitt's lymphoma
a. There is a B-cell lymphoma
b. There is a higher incidence in the black African population
c. The African type is characterised by high titres to the Epstein–Barr virus
d. The American type affects the jaw in 50% of cases
e. The survival rate is up to 60% in stage IA

24. In phaeochromocytoma
a. Paroxysmal hypertension is common
b. The blood sugar may be raised
c. There is an association with tuberose sclerosis
d. There is an association with Sipple's syndrome
e. Orthostatic hypotension is due to alpha adrenergic stimulation

25. Side-effects of anti-malignancy chemotherapy include
a. Cisplatin — ototoxicity
b. Vincristine — renal tubular damage
c. Methotrexate — liver damage
d. Daunorubicin — pulmonary fibrosis
e. Bleomycin — cystitis

Answers overleaf

21. a. True
b. True
c. True
d. True
e. True

22. a. True
b. False
c. True
d. False
e. True

23. a. True
b. True
c. True
d. False   Mainly abdominal
e. False   More than 80%

24. a. ~~False~~ *True*   Mainly orthostatic hypotension
b. True   Low or high
c. False   Association with neurofibromatosis type I
d. True
e. False   Due to beta adrenergic stimulation

25. a. True   As well as renal failure
b. False   Bone marrow failure and peripheral motor neuropathy are features
c. True
d. False   Cardiomyopathy and bone marrow failure
e. False   Pulmonary fibrosis

26. In Langerhans cell histocytosis (LCH)
a. There is proliferation of plasma cells
b. The process is not malignant
c. The type II cells have a low nuclear to cytoplasmic ratio
d. The skeleton is involved in 80% of cases
e. It may be asymptomatic

27. Recognized features of neuroblastoma include
a. Bilateral Horner's syndrome
b. Hypotension
c. Stridor
d. Epistaxis
e. Opisthomyoclonus

28. In Ewing's sarcoma
a. The usual age of presentation is less than 5 years
b. It only affects the flat bones
c. It may improve with antibiotics
d. The tumour is sensitive to radiotherapy but not to chemotherapy
e. There is a 40–60% survival rate for 3 years after surgery

29. Retinoblastoma is characterized by
a. An autosomal dominant inheritance
b. A deletion on chromosome 13
c. An association with osteosarcoma in 10% of cases
d. Calcification in 75% of cases
e. Early metastases to the brain

Answers overleaf

26. a. True
    b. False
    c. False Type I
    d. True Characterized by osteolytic lesions
    e. True

27. a. False Usually unilateral
    b. True And hypertension
    c. True Mediastinal mass
    d. True
    e. True

28. a. False More than 10 years of age
    b. False Also the long bones
    c. False
    d. False Both
    e. False Only up to 20%

29. a. True
    b. True
    c. True
    d. True
    e. False Usually localized tumour

Immunology

1. **Characteristics of the immune system in children include**
   a. IgG crosses the placenta
   b. IgA is present in low concentrations in breast-milk
   c. The thymus gland is responsible for humoral immunity
   d. Immunoglobulin levels fall progressively in the first 3 months of life
   e. High IgM levels in newborn babies may indicate postnatal infection

2. **With regard to cell-mediated immunity**
   a. Antigen-specific function is the role of T-lymphocytes
   b. It is important in protection against protozoal and fungal infection
   c. It is responsible for the delayed hypersensitivity reaction
   d. Activated T cells secrete mediators important for cellular immunity
   e. It activates the complement system

3. **The immune system in children is characterized by**
   a. A complement system producing opsonic, chemotactic reactions against infective agents
   b. The alternative complement pathway uses factors C1–9
   c. Phagocytosis is performed mainly by polymorphonuclear leukocytes
   d. Deficiency of properidin may lead to meningococcal meningitis
   e. Interleukin 1(IL-1) activates T cells to produce IL-2

4. **True or false**
   a. Defects of phagocytic function can lead to streptococcal skin infection
   b. The Chediak–Higashi syndrome is characterized by abnormal neutrophils
   c. Recurrent meningococcal infection may be due to deficiency of C5,6,7 and 8 levels
   d. Schwachman's syndrome is characterized by lymphopenia
   e. Chronic granulomatous disease has an autosomal dominant inheritance

Answers overleaf

1. a. True
    b. False   IgA is usually high in concentration
    c. False   Cellular immunity
    d. True
    e. False   If specific IgM is detected in the newborn babies it indicates intrauterine infection

2. a. True   This is a function of humoral immunity as well
    b. True
    c. True   T cells are helpers, suppressors and killers
    d. True
    e. False

3. a. True   And also neutralization of viruses
    b. False   Alternative pathway has C3,5,6,7,8 and 9
    c. False   Phagocytosis mainly by macrophages, lymphocytes and monocytes
    d. True   Factor 1 deficiency may cause severe pyogenic infection
    e. True

4. a. True
    b. True
    c. False   Properidin defects predispose to meningococcal meningitis
    d. False   Neutropenia with pancreatic insufficiency is the commonest feature of Schwachman's syndrome
    e. False   X-linked recessive inheritance

5. Features of the Wiskott–Aldrich syndrome include
a. X-Linked dominant inheritance
b. Thrombocytopenia
c. Eczema
d. A low lymphocyte count
e. Elevated IgA levels

6. In the Chediak–Higashi syndrome
a. Inheritance is autosomal recessive
b. The neutrophils contain giant cytoplasmic granules
c. It is associated with vitiligo
d. Poor opsonization is the main defect
e. There is an association with bony abnormalities

7. In Bruton's syndrome
a. Inheritance is X-linked autosomal recessive
b. It can present after the age of 5 years
c. There is no benefit from treatment with i.v. immunoglobulins
d. There may be an associated arthritis
e. Repeated ear infection is common

8. Features of chronic granulomatous disease include
a. Autosomal dominant inheritance
b. An abnormal oxidative metabolic response during phagocytosis
c. Over 90% of granulocytes react positively with the nitroblue tetrazolium (NTB) test
d. Catalase-containing bacteria are the main cause of recurrent infection
e. A bone marrow transplant is one treatment option

9. The following statements relating to severe combined immune deficiency syndrome are correct
a. It is usually inherited as X-linked recessive
b. White cell transfusions can be used in its treatment
c. The results of bone marrow transplantation are poor
d. Prenatal diagnosis is possible in 20% of cases
e. Tonsillar and thymic shadows are absent

Answers overleaf

5. a. False X-linked recessive
   b. True   Eczema and repeated ear infection are the characteristic features of Wiskott–Aldrich syndrome
   c. True
   d. False Neutrophils are low
   e. True

6. a. True   Other characteristic features of the Chediak–Higashi syndrome include recurrent infection, partial oculocutaneous albinism, photophobia and nystagmus
   b. True
   c. False
   d. False Associated with chemotactic defects
   e. False May be associated with neurological abnormalities (mental retardation, peripheral neuropathy as well as long tract and cerebellar involvement)

7. a. True
   b. True
   c. False
   d. True
   e. True   It can be an early presentation

8. a. False X-linked and autosomal recessive patients are girls
   b. True
   c. False Negative NTB test in >90% of cases
   d. True
   e. True

9. a. True   But can be autosomal recessive in 20% of cases
   b. False Leukocyte transfusion is contraindicated as the risk of GVHD is very high
   c. False The cure rate is very high and can be up to 90%
   d. True   Adenosine deaminase deficiency is the commonest defect and can be diagnosed antenatally
   e. True

10. **C1 esterase inhibitor deficiency (angioneurotic oedema) is characterized by**
    a. Abdominal pain
    b. Improves with blood transfusion
    c. Anaphylactic shock is the commonest cause of death
    d. Oedema of the face is common
    e. Danazol is the prophylactic treatment of choice

11. **The following statements relating to Kawasaki's disease are correct**
    a. There is a mortality rate of 1-2%
    b. Intravenous immunoglobulin is no more effective in treatment than aspirin alone
    c. T-helper cells are involved in the disease process
    d. It can cause myocardial infarction
    e. Steroids have no place in the treatment

Answers overleaf

10. a. True
    b. True
    c. True   Due to URT obstruction
    d. True   Urticaria is another common feature
    e. True

11. a. True   Due to coronary artery aneurysm
    b. False
    c. True
    d. True
    e. True

Nephrology

1. **The following statements relating to the physiology of body fluids and electrolytes are correct**
   a. 65% of body weight in children is water
   b. Extracellular fluid makes up 20% of body weight
   c. 1/3 of sodium is absorbed osmotically in the proximal tubule
   d. A decrease in osmolality can stimulate ADH secretion
   e. Hypovolaemia will stimulate ADH secretion

2. **The following statements about renal function in children are true**
   a. GFR reaches adult levels by the age of 1–2 years
   b. Fractional urinary excretion of sodium is low in newborn babies
   c. Urinary phosphate excretion is low throughout the growth peroid
   d. Glucose absorption occurs mainly in the proximal tubules
   e. Hydrogen ion excretion is a function of the collecting ducts

3. **Features of the congenital nephrotic syndrome include**
   a. Autosomal recessive inheritance
   b. Minimal change glomerulonephritis is a common finding
   c. A large oedematous placenta
   d. Highly selective proteinuria is pathognomonic
   e. 25% can survive the first year

4. **Infectious agents which are associated with acute glomerulonephritis include**
   a. Coxsackie virus
   b. Measles virus
   c. Rubella virus
   d. Salmonella typhi
   e. *E. Coli*

5. **Drugs known to cause haematuria include**
   a. Methicillin
   b. Heparin
   c. Sodium valproate
   d. Gold
   e. Chlorpromazine

Answers overleaf

1. a. True
   b. True   Intracellular is 40% of the total body weight
   c. False   2/3 of the water and sodium are osmotically absorbed in the proximal renal tubules
   d. False   Rises in osmolality and hypovolaemia can stimulate ADH secretion
   e. True

2. a. True
   b. False   High
   c. True
   d. True
   e. True   Distal collecting duct

3. a. True
   b. False   Microcystic change is the commonest finding
   c. True   More than 25% of the weight of the baby
   d. False   Present but not pathognomonic
   e. True   If dialysis started in the first few days of life

4. a. True   And mumps, hepatitis B
   b. True   And Echo virus, Epstein-Barr virus
   c. False
   d. True
   e. False

5. a. True   And ampicillin, penicillin
   b. True   And warfarin
   c. False
   d. True   And lead, phosphorus
   e. True

6. **Recognized causes of glomerulonephritis with hypocomplementaemia include**
   a. Post-streptococcal glomerulonephritis
   b. Systemic lupus erythematosus (SLE)
   c. Membranous glomerulonephritis
   d. Bacterial endocarditis
   e. Henoch–Schonlein nephritis

7. **The following statements relating to calcium metabolism are correct**
   a. Ionized calcium is not functionally active
   b. Hypercalcaemia may cause constipation
   c. Thiazide diuretics can be used in the treatment of hypercalcaemia
   d. Alkalosis may reduce ionized calcium with no symptoms of hypocalcaemia
   e. Chvostek's sign is carpopedal spasm and Trousseau's sign is contraction of the facial muscles

8. **Common causes of proteinuria of more than 10 g/24 h include**
   a. Orthostatic proteinuria
   b. Post-streptococcal glomerulonephritis
   c. Chronic lead poisoning
   d. Chronic renal failure
   e. Minimal change nephrotic syndrome

9. **Common histopathological changes in nephrotic syndrome include**
   a. Membranoproliferative glomerulonephritis in 50% of cases
   b. Mesangial-proliferative glomerulonephritis in more than 5% of cases
   c. Focal and segmental glomerulosclerosis in 10% of cases
   d. Rapidly progressive crescentic glomerulonephritis
   e. Minimal change glomerulonephritis in 85% of cases

Answers overleaf

6. a. True   Especially following throat infection
   b. True   This is mainly due to immune complex reaction
   c. False   This may cause nephrotic syndrome
   d. True   Due to immune complex reaction
   e. False

7. a. False   This is the only functional form of active calcium
   b. True   And polyuria
   c. False   Frusemide. Thiazides may cause hypercalcaemia
   d. True
   e. False   Chvostek's sign is the contraction of facial muscle on tapping the mandibular joints. Trousseau's sign is the carpopedal spasm of fingers on tapping the small muscles of the hand

8. a. False   Bengin proteinuria of < 1 g/24 h
   b. False
   c. True   And other causes of nephrotic syndrome
   d. False   Proteinuria may become heavy during the end stages of renal failure
   e. True   This is the commonest cause of heavy proteinuria

9. a. False   In < 2%
   b. True   And characterized by a diffuse increase in mesangial cells and matrix. 50-60% of patients respond to steroids
   c. True   20% of these patients respond to steroids but it leads to end-stage renal failure in most patients
   d. False   Below 1%
   e. True   This is the commonest cause

10. **Recognized causes of acute glomerulonephritis are**
    a. Minimal change glomerulonephritis
    b. SLE
    c. Polyarteritis nodosa
    d. Anti-basement membrane antibody glomerulonephritis
    e. Streptococcal skin infection

11. **Characteristic features of Berger's disease include**
    a. Autosomal dominant inheritance
    b. Deposition of C3 and IgA in the mesangium
    c. A preceding upper respiratory tract infection in most cases
    d. The majority progress to chronic renal failure after 10 years
    e. Recurrent haematuria is pathognomonic

12. **The following are normal contents of urine**
    a. < 4 white cells
    b. Granular casts
    c. White cell casts
    d. Epithelial cells
    e. Hexagonal crystals

13. **Histopathological changes in the kidneys in systemic lupus erythromatosis include**
    a. Membranous lupus nephritis
    b. Focal proliferative lupus nephritis
    c. Mesangial lupus nephritis
    d. 'Wire loop' lesions
    e. Normal kidneys

14. **Histopathological findings in the kidneys in diabetes mellitus include**
    a. Kimmelstiel–Wilson changes
    b. Glomerular basement membrane thickening
    c. Proliferative glomerulonephritis
    d. Aneurysms of the renal vessels
    e. Mesangial sclerosis

Answers overleaf

10. a. False   Causes nephrotic syndrome
     b. True   Both nephrotic and nephritic syndrome
     c. True
     d. True   Goodpasture's syndrome characterized by
                 pulmonary haemorrhage and glomerulonephritis
                 associated with antibodies against lung and
                 glomerular basement membrane
     e. True

11. a. False   The familial occurence is rare
     b. True
     c. False
     d. False   This happens in males in Alport's syndrome
     e. False   Recurrent haematuria can be familial

12. a. True
     b. True   Red cell casts in glomerulonephritis
     c. False   Commonly associated with infection and
                 malignancy
     d. True
     e. False   Found in cystinuria

13. a. True   With proteinuria
     b. False   Diffuse proliferative nephritis
     c. True   With mild proteinuria
     d. True   With high blood pressure, nephrotic syndrome
                 and loss of renal function
     e. True

14. a. True   The commonest glomerular lesions associated
                 with DM
     b. True
     c. False   Can be associated with Henoch–Schonlein
                 purpura
     d. False   May be associated with polyarteritis nodosa
     e. True

15. **The following statements about renal as opposed to pre-renal failure are correct**
    a.   Urinary Na >20 mmol/l
    b.   Urine osmolality <400 mosmol/kg water
    c.   Urine plasma urea: ratio is >5
    d.   Fractional excretion of sodium (FENa %) $<1\%$
    e.   Plasma creatinine greater than 60 μmol/l

16. **Common causes of chronic renal failure include**
    a.   Reflux nephropathy
    b.   Glomerulonephritis
    c.   Congenital abnormalities
    d.   Urinary tract infection
    e.   Renal calculi

17. **The following statements about proximal renal tubular acidosis are correct**
    a.   Urine pH is >6
    b.   Can be familial
    c.   The net excretion of acid is normal
    d.   Nephrocalcinosis may occur
    e.   It responds to treatment with a low dose of bicarbonate

18. **Common causes of Fanconi's syndrome include**
    a.   Galactosaemia
    b.   Lowe's syndrome
    c.   Idiopathic
    d.   Cystinosis
    e.   Lead poisoning

19. **Characteristic features of Bartter's syndrome include**
    a.   Hypoaldosteronism
    b.   Hypokalaemia
    c.   High blood pressure
    d.   Hypertrophy of the juxta-glomerular apparatus
    e.   Indomethacin is the treatment of choice

Answers overleaf

15. a. True
  b. True
  c. True
  d. False   More than 1%
  e. False   Creatinine elevated in both conditions

16. a. True   In 70%
  b. True
  c. False   Not common
  d. False   Only if associated with vesico-ureteric reflux
  e. False

17. a. False   Urine pH is more than 6 in the presence of
          acidosis
  b. True   Hypokalaemia, urine pH below 5, metabolic
          acidosis, aminoaciduria, hyperphosphaturia,
          glycosuria and failure to thrive are other features
          of proximal renal tubular acidosis (type 2 RTA)
  c. True
  d. False   In distal renal tubular acidosis
  e. True

18. a. False
  b. True
  c. True
  d. True
  e. False

19. a. False   Hyperaldosteronism with high serum renin level
          which increases the renal exchange of sodium for
          potassium or hydrogen ion in the distal tubule
          resulting in hypokalaemic alkalosis
  b. True   And hyponatraemia
  c. False   Normal blood pressure
  d. True
  e. True   Oral potassium supplements and the aldosterone
          antagonist spironolactone can be used in
          treatment

20. True or false
   a. Uric acid stones are radio-opaque
   b. Cystine stones are caused by renal tubular acidosis
   c. Magnesium ammonium phosphate stones are radiopaque
   d. Primary oxalosis is associated with radiopaque stones
   e. Immobilization can cause magnesium ammonium phosphate stones

Answers overleaf

20. a. False
    b. False   More commonly associated with cystinuria
    c. True
    d. True
    e. False   Can cause calcium phosphate stones

Neurology

1. **Characteristic features of lower motor neurone lesions include**
   a. An increase in tone
   b. Wasting of the affected muscles
   c. Loss of abdominal reflexes
   d. Clonus
   e. An extensor plantar reflex

2. **Recognized signs of an extrapyramidal tract lesion include**
   a. Absence of reflexes
   b. Dysarthria
   c. Fibrillation
   d. 'Cog wheel rigidity'
   e. Hypotonia

3. **Sensory lesions in the anterolateral columns of the spinal cord are characterized by**
   a. Loss of touch sensation ipsilaterally
   b. Loss of pain sensation contralaterally
   c. Vibration sense is abolished ipsilaterally below the lesion
   d. Exquisite pain on the opposite side
   e. Astereognosis

4. **An extensor plantar reflex commonly occurs in**
   a. Infants
   b. After a generalized convulsions
   c. Quadriplegic cerebral palsy
   d. A lower motor neurone lesion
   e. Comatose children

5. **The following statements relating to bladder control are correct**
   a. The sympathetic fibres arise from the 3rd and 4th lumbar segments
   b. Sympathetic fibres relax the bladder wall
   c. Pelvic nerves via S2,3 and 4 relax the sphincters
   d. Somatic nerves via S2,3 and 4 relax the external sphincter of the urethra
   e. Lesions of the anterior sacral nerve roots cause an atonic bladder

Answers overleaf

1. a. False   Upper motor neurone lesion
    b. True
    c. False
    d. False
    e. False

2. a. False   Occurs with lower motor neurone lesions
    b. True
    c. False   Occurs with lower motor neurone lesions
    d. True
    e. True

3. a. True
    b. True
    c. False   Occurs with posterior column lesions
    d. False   Occurs with thalamic lesions
    e. False

4. a. True
    b. True
    c. True   And diplegic and hemiplegic cerebral palsy
    d. False   Upper motor neurone lesion
    e. True

5. a. False   From lumbar segments 1 and 2
    b. True   And contract the sphincters
    c. True   And contract the bladder wall
    d. False   Contracts the external sphincter of the urethra
    e. True

6. **The clinical manifestations of lesions of the visual pathway include**
   a. Optic nerve — no light reflex
   b. Optic chiasm — quadrantic hemianopia
   c. Optic tracts — homonymous hemianopia
   d. Optic radiation (temporal) — upper quadrant homonymous hemianopia
   e. Occipital cortex — homonymous hemianopia

7. **Lesions in the parietal lobes are characterized by**
   a. Apraxia
   b. Déja vu phenomena
   c. Perceptual rivalry
   d. Auditory hallucinations
   e. Agnosia

8. **Proprioceptive sensory loss in children can be due to**
   a. The Guillain–Barre syndrome
   b. Friedreich's ataxia
   c. Charcot–Marie–Tooth disease
   d. Vincristine therapy
   e. Medulloblastoma

9. **Common causes of a bilateral facial nerve palsy in children include**
   a. Moebius' syndrome
   b. Bell's palsy
   c. Guillain–Barre syndrome
   d. Hypertension
   e. Ramsay–Hunt syndrome

10. **Hyper-reflexia is a characteristic feature of**
    a. Encephalitis
    b. Duchenne muscular dystrophy
    c. Cerebral palsy
    d. Spinal lesions
    e. Werdnig–Hoffmann disease

Answers overleaf

6. a. True   And loss of vision in the affected eye
    b. True
    c. True
    d. True
    e. True

7. a. True
    b. False   Temporal lobes
    c. True   The brain ignores the stimulus on the side contralateral to the parietal lobe
    d. False   Temporal lobes
    e. True

8. a. True   And lower motor neurone signs
    b. True   As well as cerebellar, upper motor and corticospinal signs
    c. True
    d. True   And peripheral neuropathy
    e. False

9. a. True
    b. False
    c. True
    d. False   This usually causes a unilateral facial nerve palsy
    e. False   This is due to middle ear infection with herpes zoster and usually affects the geniculate body of the facial nerve nuclei

10. a. True
    b. False
    c. True
    d. True   Occurs in the acute stages
    e. False   Absence of reflexes is due to involvement of anterior horn cells of the spinal cord

11. **CSF lymphocytosis is commonly associated with**
    a. Kawasaki's disease
    b. Leptospirosis
    c. Guillain–Barré syndrome
    d. Cerebral abscess
    e. Cryptococcal infection

12. **Acute cerebellar ataxia is associated with the following conditions**
    a. astrocytomas
    b. Phenytoin toxicity
    c. Migraine
    d. Chicken-pox infection
    e. Ataxia telangiectasia

13. **The following muscles are supplied by the following nerves**
    a. Trapezius — Accessory nerve
    b. Interossei — Ulnar nerve
    c. Tibialis anterior — peroneal nerve
    d. Brachioradialis — Median nerve
    e. Abductor pollicis brevis — ulnar nerve

14. **Clinical features of an absent corpus collosum include**
    a. Normal intelligence
    b. An association with colobomata of the retina
    c. Blindness
    d. Hemihypsarrhythmia on EEG
    e. Bilateral Erb's palsy

15. **The following statements relating to normal CSF are correct**
    a. The rate of production is 0.5–1 ml/min
    b. Hypothermia reduces production
    c. It leaves the ventricular system through the foramen of Monro
    d. It returns to the venous sinuses via the choroid plexuses
    e. Normal CSF pressure is 20–30 cmHg

Answers overleaf

11. a. False   Not commonly
    b. True
    c. True   With normal sugar and high protein
    d. False   May have a high protein level
    e. True

12. a. True
    b. True
    c. True
    d. True
    e. False   Chronic ataxia with bulbar telangiectasia are the commonest features. Low IgM and high IgA, high alpha-fetoprotein are other features of this condition

13. a. True   As well as the sternomastoid muscle
    b. True
    c. True
    d. False   By the radial nerve
    e. False   By the median nerve

14. a. True
    b. True   This is associated with the Aicardi syndrome which is characterized by absence of the corpus callosum
    c. False
    d. True   Aicardi syndrome
    e. False   Arnold–Chiari malformation

15. a. False   Usually 2–3 ml/min from choroid plexuses in the lateral, third and fourth ventricles
    b. True
    c. False   Through the aqueduct of Sylvius in the roof of fourth ventricle
    d. False   By the arachnoid villi
    e. False   Up to 5–15 cmHg with the patient lying on one side

16. Non-communicating hydrocephalus may be due to
a. Obstruction of the aqueduct of Sylvius
b. Obstruction of the basal cisterns
c. Obstruction of the foramen of Munroe
d. Obstruction of the outlet of the lateral ventricles
e. Arachnoiditis

17. Characteristic features of benign intracranial hypertension include
a. Papilloedema
b. Upper motor neurone signs
c. VIth nerve palsy
d. Frontal headache
e. Large ventricles on CT scan of the head

18. Drugs which are effective in the treatment of infantile spasms include
a. Carbamazepine
b. ACTH
c. Vigabatrin
d. Sodium valproate
e. Clonazepam

19. The following are features of Petit mal epilepsy
a. Asymmetrical 3 cps (cycles per second) of generalized spike-wave complexes on EEG
b. It may be accompanied by automatism
c. Onset is commonly between the ages of 11–13 years
d. A duration of more than 30 seconds is abnormal
e. Sodium valproate will control attacks in more than 80% of cases

20. Drugs which inhibit phenytoin metabolism include
a. Chloramphenicol
b. Nitrazepam
c. Sodium valproate
d. Carbamazepine
e. Isoniazid

Answers overleaf

16. a. True
  b. False Communicating hydrocephalus
  c. True And Arnold–Chiari malformation
  d. True
  e. False

17. a. True As well as headache
  b. False None
  c. True Not common
  d. False Generalized headache
  e. False Are small or normal

18. a. False Mainly for simple and complex partial seizures
  b. True And prednisolone
  c. True
  d. True
  e. True

19. a. False Symmetrical
  b. True
  c. False Age of onset 3–9 years (peak 4–8)
  d. True Over 90% of seizures last between 5 and 15 seconds
  e. True

20. a. True
  b. False
  c. True
  d. False
  e. True

21. Characteristic features of Duchenne muscular dystrophy (DMD) include
a. Intelligence is always normal
b. Delay in walking and talking has no relation to the DMD
c. An increased level of umbilical cord creatinine kinase is diagnostic
d. A decrease in action potential on EMG is diagnostic
e. A Q-wave is found in all ECG chest leads in older patients

22. Dystrophia myotonica is characterized by
a. Autosomal dominant inheritance
b. Muscle fibrillation
c. Mental retardation
d. Infertility
e. Diabetes mellitus

23. Spinal muscle atrophy is characterized by
a. Alertness
b. Absent reflexes
c. Cataracts
d. A decrease in motor nerve conduction velocity
e. Clubfeet

24. Diagnostic features of type I neurofibromatosis include
a. Five or more café-au-lait spots
b. Adenoma sebaceum
c. Inguinal freckling
d. Phacomata
e. Bilateral acoustic neuroma

25. Recognized features of a neuro-degenerative disorder in children include
a. Progressive loss of vision
b. Normal intelligence
c. Feeding difficulties
d. Seizures
e. Lower motor neurone signs

Answers overleaf

21. a. False   Mental retardation occurs in about 10–30% of cases
    b. False   This could be the earliest manifestation.
    c. False   Not a reliable test. The diagnostic test is a muscle biopsy which is characterized by variable sizes of muscle fibres, adipose tissue and abnormal nuclei of the muscle fibres
    d. False
    e. True   Cardiomyopathy is a constant feature and some patients will die early of severe cardiomyopathy

22. a. True   Diagnostic tests are muscle biopsy and EMG
    b. False   Common with spinal muscular atrophy
    c. True   In 50% of cases
    d. True   And cataract
    e. True   Thyroid and adrenal function should be assessed as well as immunoglobulins and ECG

23. a. True   And fasciculation of the tongue or other muscles
    b. True
    c. False
    d. False   Normal
    e. False

24. a. True   Of more than 5 mm in size in prepubertal patients and more than five cafe-au-lait spots over 15 mm in post-pubertal patients
    b. False
    c. True
    d. False
    e. False   This is a characteristic feature of NF-2

25. a. True   As well as speech, and developmental skills which have been acquired in previous years
    b. False
    c. True
    d. True
    e. False   Upper motor neurone signs

26. **Absent knee jerks and extensor plantar reflexes in children are characteristic of**
    a. Cord compression at L4/5
    b. Friedreich's ataxia
    c. Metachromatic leucodystrophy
    d. Vitamin B_{12} deficiency
    e. Cerebral palsy

27. **Characteristic features of limb girdle muscular dystrophy include**
    a. Autosomal dominant inheritance
    b. There may be associated hypertrophy of the calf muscles
    c. Death in the late twenties
    d. Mental retardation
    e. Winging of the scapula

28. **Proximal muscle weakness occurs in**
    a. Thyrotoxicosis
    b. Hypothyroidism
    c. Cushing's disease
    d. Conn's syndrome
    e. Familial hypokalaemic periodic paralysis

29. **Recognized features of dermatomyositis include**
    a. A proximal symmetrical weakness
    b. Normal creatinine kinase levels
    c. Vasculopathy on muscle biopsy
    d. It affects boys more than girls
    e. 90% respond to steroids

30. **Drugs which may precipitate myasthenia gravis include**
    a. Succinylcholine
    b. Kanamycin
    c. Atropine
    d. Streptomycin
    e. Pyridostigmine

Answers overleaf

26. a. False   L3/4 lesion
    b. True
    c. True
    d. True   In chronic deficiency
    e. False

27. a. False   Autosomal recessive. Occasionally autosomal dominant
    b. True
    c. False
    d. False   Intelligence is normal
    e. False   Usually associated with facio-scapulo-humoral muscle atrophy

28. a. True
    b. True   And hyperthyroidism
    c. True
    d. True
    e. True

29. a. True   Which is progressive
    b. False   CK and other muscle enzymes are elevated
    c. True   And ischaemic myopathy. Multifocal EMG changes
    d. False   More common in girls
    e. True

30. a. True
    b. True   And other aminoglycosides
    c. False
    d. True
    e. False   This is used in the treatment of myasthenia gravis

31. **Characteristic features of hereditary motor sensory neuropathy type I (HMSN I) include**
  a. Autosomal dominant inheritance
  b. Argyll–Robertson pupils
  c. It usually presents as early as five years of age
  d. Pes cavus
  e. Proprioceptive sensation is affected

Answer   overleaf

31. a. True
b. False
c. False   Asymptomatic until late childhood or early adolescence. The peroneal and tibial nerves are the earliest and most severely affected. Child becomes clumsy and trips easily
d. True
e. True   And vibration sensation

Child psychiatry

1. **Characteristic features of infantile autism include**
   a. Echolalia
   b. Obsessive patterns of behaviour
   c. Onset usually after the age of 30 months
   d. The risk of recurrence is high in the same family
   e. It is more common in children with parents who have schizoid personalities

2. **Features of depressive illness in adolescence include**
   a. Truancy
   b. Sleep disturbance
   c. Alcohol and drug abuse
   d. A positive family history
   e. Self harm

3. **The following statements relating to suicide in adolescence are correct**
   a. It is more common in females than males
   b. Drug overdose is the commonest method used by boys
   c. Announcing an intention to commit suicide is to be taken more seriously than leaving a suicide note
   d. Previous unsuccessful attempts require close observation
   e. Chronically ill children are more likely to commit suicide

4. **Hormonal changes in anorexia nervosa include**
   a. Low GH
   b. Low LH and FSH
   c. High cortisol
   d. High somatomedin
   e. Low TSH

5. **True or false relating to anorexia nervosa**
   a. ESR is commonly low
   b. Constipation is very common
   c. Blood and urine nitrogen levels are low
   d. Hypochloraemic alkalosis is not common
   e. There is an increased susceptibility to infection

Answers overleaf

1. a. True   And avoidance of eye to eye contact
     b. True
     c. False   Usual onset is under the age of 30 months
     d. False   It is very common for only one child in the family
              to be affected
     e. False   There is no relation between schizoid personality
              and autism in the family

2. a. True
     b. True
     c. True
     d. True
     e. True

3. a. True
     b. False   Drugs are most commonly used by girls while
              violent methods are used more commonly by boys
     c. False   Leaving a suicidal note is more serious than
              announcing an intent
     d. True   They should be kept under close observation
     e. True

4. a. False   High or normal
     b. True
     c. True
     d. False   Low
     e. False   TSH normal and T3 and T4 are low

5. a. True
     b. True
     c. False   Normal or high
     d. True   Commonly associated with bulimia
     e. False

6. Common side-effects of anti-depressant drugs include
   a. Weight gain
   b. A prolonged P-R interval on ECG
   c. Hypertension
   d. Orthostatic hypotension
   e. A dry mouth

7. Features of depressed school-age children are
   a. Panic-like behaviour
   b. Easy tears
   c. Vegetative symptoms
   d. Withdrawal
   e. Staring into space

8. Side-effects of chlorpromazine include
   a. Abdominal pain
   b. Dyskinesia
   c. Contact sensitivity
   d. Worsening of tics
   e. Constipation

9. The following are recognized features of lithium toxicity
   a. Dysarthria
   b. Ataxia
   c. Coarse tremor
   d. Neuromuscular irritability
   e. Neonatal goitre

10. The following drugs can block the action of anti-depressants
   a. Haloperidol
   b. Guanethidine
   c. Propranolol
   d. Reserpine
   e. Griseofulvin

Answers overleaf

6. a. False   Weight loss is the commonest side-effect
    b. True
    c. False
    d. True
    e. True

7. a. True
    b. True
    c. True   Eating and sleeping disorders are common
    d. True
    e. False

8. a. False
    b. True   Other side-effect of chlorpromazine treatment include: extra-pyramidal signs and postural hypotension
    c. True
    d. False   This is a side-effect of stimulant drugs
    e. True

9. a. True   Other side-effects include: nausea, vomiting, tremor, myopathy, polyuria and cardio-respiratory symptoms
    b. True
    c. True
    d. True
    e. True

10. a. True
    b. False
    c. True
    d. True
    e. True

11. Which of the following drugs have anti-cholinergic side-effects
   a. Desipramine hydrochloride
   b. Nortriptyline
   c. Atropine
   d. Lithium
   e. Carbamazepine

Answer overleaf

11. a. True
    b. True
    c. True
    d. False
    e. False

Infectious diseases

1. **The following are RNA viruses**
   a. Varicella zoster
   b. Measles
   c. Parvovirus
   d. Retrovirus
   e. Hepatitis A virus

2. **The following are DNA double-stranded viruses**
   a. Rotavirus
   b. Papovavirus
   c. Adenovirus
   d. Hepatitis B virus
   e. Retroviruses

3. **Vaccines composed of live or attenuated organisms include**
   a. Haemophilus influenzae b
   b. Measles
   c. BCG
   d. Tetanus
   e. Pertussis

4. **Gram-negative cocci bacteria include**
   a. *Escherichia coli*
   b. *Neisseria meningitidis*
   c. *Streptococcus pyogenes*
   d. *Klebsiella pneumoniae*
   e. *Pseudomonas aeruginosa*

5. **Bloody diarrhoea can be caused by the following agents**
   a. *Vibrio cholera*
   b. *Shigella flexneri*
   c. *Amoebic dysentery*
   d. *Escherichia coli*
   e. *Salmonella typhi*

Answers overleaf

1. a. False   This is a DNA double-stranded virus of the herpes family
    b. True   This is an RNA single-stranded virus of the paramyxo family
    c. False   This is a DNA single-stranded virus
    d. True   This is an RNA single-stranded virus responsible for AIDS and related disorders
    e. True   This is an RNA single-stranded virus of the picorna family

2. a. False   Double-stranded RNA viruses
    b. True
    c. True
    d. True   Hepatitis A is an RNA virus
    e. False   This is an RNA single-stranded virus

3. a. False   Its pre-capsule component
    b. True
    c. True
    d. False   Toxoid
    e. False   This is an inactivated vaccine.

4. a. False   Gram-negative bacilli
    b. True
    c. False   Gram-positive cocci
    d. False   Gram-negative bacilli
    e. False   Gram-negative rods

5. a. False   Watery diarrhoea
    b. True
    c. True
    d. False   Watery diarrhoea
    e. True   And para-typhi

6. **Drugs used in the treatment of leprosy include**
   a. Dapsone
   b. Rifampicin
   c. Chloroquine
   e. Thalidomide
   e. Prednisolone

7. **Characteristic features of leptospirosis (Weil's disease) include**
   a. Jaundice
   b. Rigors
   c. Muscle pains
   d. Conjunctivitis
   e. Albuminuria

8. **Complications which may follow varicella infection (chicken-pox) include**
   a. Thrombocytopenia
   b. Diffuse nodular infiltration on chest X-ray
   c. The Ramsay–Hunt syndrome
   d. Myocarditis
   e. Reye's syndrome

9. **Characteristic features of yellow fever include**
   a. Transmission by mosquitoes
   b. A tendency to bleed
   c. An adenovirus as the causative agent
   d. Bradycardia
   e. Responds to treatment with acyclovir

10. **The following statements relating to hepatitis B virus infection are correct**
    a. It is an RNA virus
    b. Patients with HBe antigen are not infectious
    c. HBsAg can be demonstrated in saliva
    d. The incubation period is 2–6 weeks
    e. HBc-antibodies indicate protection against future infection with HB

Answers overleaf

6. a. True
b. True
c. True
d. True
e. True

7. a. True
b. False
c. True
d. True
e. True

8. a. True
b. True   And encephalitis and ataxia
c. False   This is a herpes zozster infection of the geniculate ganglia
d. True
e. True

9. a. True   *Aedes aegypti* mosquito
b. True   As well as fever, chills, headache and backache
c. False   Togavirus
d. True
e. False   No specific treatment

10. a. False   DNA virus
b. False
c. True   And stool
d. False   2–5 months
e. False   This with HBsAg indicates chronic asymptomatic carriers

11. **Characteristic features of poliomyelitis virus infection include**
   a. A motor neuropathy
   b. Neural lesions occur in the white matter
   c. Constipation as a frequent finding
   d. Muscle pain
   e. Reflexes are normal in the early stages

12. **Features of human immunodeficiency virus (HIV) include**
   a. It is an RNA enterovirus
   b. There is reverse transcriptase to DNA
   c. High plasma levels of virus are found in HIV positive patients
   d. It is transmitted by breast feeding
   e. It is usually attached to CD4 (T-helper) cells

13. **Diagnostic tests for HIV infection in infants include**
   a. Hypergammaglobulinaemia
   b. A positive HIV-antibody titre
   c. A low CD4:CD8 ratio
   d. P24 antigenaemia
   e. Positive PCR for HIV-1 DNA

14. **Characteristic features of Rickettsial infections include**
   a. Vasculitis
   b. Rashes
   c. The direct fluorescent antibody test is always positive
   d. It responds to treatment with tetracycline
   e. The Weil–Felix test is diagnostic

15. **Intracellular protozoan infections include**
   a. Sporozoites in malaria
   b. Trophozoites in malaria
   c. Leishmaniasis
   d. Toxoplasmosis
   e. American trypanosomiasis

Answers overleaf

11. a. True   No sensory neuropathy
    b. True   Mainly affects anterior horn cells
    c. True
    d. True
    e. True   And signs of a lower motor neurone lesion later

12. a. False   RNA retrovirus
    b. True
    c. False
    d. True
    e. True

13. a. False   There is hypergammaglobulinaemia associated with HIV infection but it is not diagnostic
    b. False   After 18 months of age is diagnostic
    c. False   Not diagnostic
    d. True
    e. True

14. a. True   Pneumonia and gastro-enteritis are other features
    b. False   Fever is common but rashes are classic
    c. False   In 50% of cases
    d. True   Chloramphenicol and doxycycline are also curative drugs
    e. False   Not a specific test, ELISA is more specific

15. a. False   Pre-erythrocytic phase
    b. True
    c. True   In macrophages
    d. True
    e. False   Blood and lymphatic fluid

16. Cryptococcus neoformans
   a. Is a yeast
   b. The dog is the usual host
   c. Can cause cystic lesions
   d. Griseofulvin is an effective treatment
   e. Rarely causes hearing loss

 The following statements relating to malaria infection are correct
   a. It can be transmitted by the male anopheles mosquitoes
   b. Quartan malaria is caused by *P. Vivax*
   c. A vaccine is not yet available
   d. IgG specific antibodies are common in children
   e. Resistance to current therapy is most common in East Africa

Answers overleaf

16. a. True Occurs usually as an opportunistic infection in an immunocompromised host
  b. False Birds, particularly pigeons
  c. True In the lungs
  d. False I.V. Amphotericin B plus flucytosine are the commonly used drugs for treating pulmonary or cryptococcal meningitis
  e. False Up to 40% of survivors following cryptococcal meningitis have a residual neurological defect (hearing loss, visual problems, cranial nerve damage and personality changes)

17. a. False Female
  b. False *P. malariae*
  c. False New vaccine was developed in Colombia and is available now with the help of WHO
  d. False IgM specific antibodies
  e. False South-East Asia

Dermatology

1. **The following statements relating to normal skin in children are correct**
   a. It makes up 25% of body weight
   b. The epidermis is derived from ectoderm
   c. The dermis is derived from endoderm
   d. Keratinocytes are located in the dermis
   e. Melanocytes are located in the epidermis

2. **Koebner's phenomena may be seen in**
   a. Viral warts
   b. Eczema
   c. Juvenile chronic arthritis
   d. Psoriasis
   e. Lichen planus

3. **Leg ulcers are a recognized feature of**
   a. Zinc deficiency
   b. Sickle cell anaemia
   c. Leishmaniasis
   d. Crohn's disease
   e. Epidermolysis bullosa

4. **There is an association between intracranial calcification and skin lesions in**
   a. Craniopharyngioma
   b. Tuberose sclerosis
   c. Neurofibromatosis
   d. Sturge–Weber syndrome
   e. Primary hypoparathyroidism

5. **Itching is a common manifestation of**
   a. Lichen planus
   b. Psoriasis
   c. Seborrheic dermatitis
   d. Pityriasis alba
   e. Alopecia totalis

Answers overleaf

1. a. False   Up to 15% of body weight
    b. True
    c. False   From mesoderm
    d. False   located in epidermis with blood vessels, nerve ending and hair follicles
    e. True

2. a. True
    b. False
    c. False
    d. True
    e. True

3. a. False   This is usually associated with dermatitis arround the mouth and genitalia
    b. True
    c. True
    d. True   As well as ulccrative colitis (pyoderma gangrenosum)
    e. True

4. a. False
    b. True
    c. False
    d. True   This is called 'tram line' calcification
    e. True

5. a. True
    b. False   Very rarely associated with pruritis
    c. False
    d. False   Pityriasis versicolor can cause itching
    e. False   Ringworm infection may cause itching

6. Blue sclera are a manifestation of
   a. Ehler–Danlos syndrome
   b. Marfan's syndrome
   c. Incontentia pigmenti
   d. Achondroplasia
   e. CHARGE syndrome

7. Telangiectasia are characteristic of
   a. Liver disease
   b. Nephrotic syndrome
   c. Renal disease
   d. Steroid therapy
   e. Osler–Weber–Rendu syndrome

8. Common causes of erythema nodosum include
   a. *Mycoplasma pneumoniae*
   b. Chlamydial infection
   c. Herpes simplex
   d. Tuberculosis
   e. Crohn's disease

9. Common causes of erythema multiforme include
   a. Streptococcal infection
   b. *Mycoplasma pneumoniae*
   c. Sulphonamides
   d. Herpes virus
   e. Leukaemia

10. Disorders associated with blisters include
   a. Incontinentia pigmenti
   b. Lichen planus
   c. Erythema multiforme
   d. Barbiturate poisoning
   e. Ichthyosis vulgaris

Answers overleaf

6. a. True   Associated with hyperelastic skin, hyper-extendable joints and tissue paper scars
   b. True
   c. True   X-linked dominant disease with mental retardation and epilepsy
   d. False   Osteogenesis imperfecta is usually associated with blue sclera
   e. False   CHARGE associations are colobomas, heart defect, anal atresia, renal anomalies, growth and mental deficiency and ear anomalies

7. a. True   Spider naevi
   b. False
   c. False
   d. True
   e. True   Also called hereditary haemorrhagic telangiectasia

8. a. True
   b. False
   c. False   A rare cause
   d. True
   e. True   And ulcerative colitis

9. a. False   Not common
   b. True
   c. True
   d. True
   e. False   Not common

10. a. True
   b. True
   c. True
   d. True
   e. False

11. Hypomelanosis may be seen in the following condition
   a. Leopard syndrome
   b. Phenylketonuria
   c. Chloroquine treatment
   e. Kwashiorkor
   e. Malignant melanoma

12. Drugs which can cause photosensitivity include
   a. Phenothiazines
   b. Frusemide
   c. Erythromycin
   d. Sulphonamides
   e. Sulphonylureas

13. Patchy alopecia without scarring can be associated with
   a. Tinea capitis
   b. Scleroderma
   c. Alopecia areata
   d. Lichen planus
   e. Psoriasis

14. Drugs which may cause hypertrichosis include
   a. Diazoxide
   b. Steroids
   c. Sulphonamides
   d. Sodium valproate
   e. Cyclosporin A

Answers overleaf

11. a. False   Hypermelanosis and is characterised by
                  pulmonary stenosis, basal-cell nevi, broad
                  facies and rib abnormalities
     b. True
     c. True
     d. False   Hypermelanosis
     e. True

12. a. True
     b. False
     c. False
     d. True
     e. True

13. a. True
     b. False
     c. True
     d. False   This can cause scarring alopecia
     e. True

14. a. True
     b. True
     c. False
     d. False
     e. True

Bone and joint diseases

1. **The following statements relating to normal synovial fluid are correct**
   a. It is colourless
   b. There are more polymorphonuclear cells than lymphocytes
   c. The viscosity is high
   d. The glucose level is 2/3 that of the blood glucose level
   e. The presence of fibrin indicates inflammation

2. **Features of Still's disease include**
   a. Remittent fever
   b. An age of onset between 5 and 10 years of age
   c. The cervical joints are not involved
   d. Micrognathia
   e. Leucocytosis

3. **Common features of polyarticular JCA include**
   a. New bone formation
   b. A positive ANF (anti-nuclear factor)
   c. Systemic features are diagnostic
   d. It is more common in girls
   e. The cervical spine is involved in half the cases over 5 years of age

4. **Common causes of limping in a 10-year-old child include**
   a. Transient synovitis
   b. Perthe's disease
   c. JCA (juvenile chronic arthritis)
   d. Muscle disease
   e. Leukaemia

5. **The following statements relating to rheumatoid factor are correct**
   a. It is an antibody to abnormal IgG
   b. It is positive in endocarditis
   c. It is of the IgM class of antibodies
   d. It is positive in 10% cases of JCA
   e. It is positive in polyarteritis nodosa

Answers overleaf

1. a. True
    b. False   Mainly lymphocytes
    c. True
    d. False   It is the same as the blood sugar level
    e. True

2. a. True
    b. False   Common in children of 5 years or below
    c. False
    d. True
    e. True   An ESR of over 100 mm per hour, thrombocythaemia, hypergammaglobulinaemia and leucocytosis are supportive laboratory data for the diagnosis of Still's disease

3. a. True
    b. False   This is a feature of pauciarticular JCA
    c. False   Systemic features are not marked
    d. True
    e. True

4. a. True   Trauma is another cause
    b. True   Slipped femoral epiphysis can cause limping in the obese child
    c. True
    d. False
    e. False   Not a common cause

5. a. False   It is an antibody to normal IgG
    b. True   Rheumatoid factor is positive in SLE, systemic sclerosis, 4% of the normal population and mixed connective tissue disease
    c. True
    d. True
    e. False

6. **The following immunological phenomena can occur with SLE**
   a. Antibodies to RNA nucleoprotein are found in up to 80% of cases
   b. Antibodies to ribonucleoprotein
   c. Antibodies to single-stranded DNA
   d. ANF is positive in most cases
   e. Rheumatoid factor is positive in 70% of cases

7. **The biochemistry of rickets is characterized by**
   a. Hypocalcaemia
   b. High alkaline phosphatase levels
   c. A reduction in the plasma level of 25-hydroxycholecalciferol as the first biochemical abnormality
   d. A high urinary phosphate concentration
   e. Amino-aciduria

8. **Premature craniosynostenosis occurs in the following conditions**
   a. Neonatal rickets
   b. Cruzon's syndrome (craniofacial dysostosis)
   c. Apert's syndrome (acrocephalosyndactyly)
   d. Frontal plagiocephaly
   e. Craniocleidodysostosis

9. **In osteogenesis imperfecta**
   a. Blue sclera are diagnostic
   b. The autosomal recessive type may be lethal in the neonatal period
   c. Conductive hearing loss (otosclerosis) may occur
   d. Patients have normal teeth
   e. A 'telephone receiver' shape of the femur bone on X-ray is diagnostic

10. **Common causes of sclerotic bone lesions include**
    a. Langerhans histocytic disease
    b. Bone tumours
    c. Leukaemia
    d. McCune–Albright syndrome
    e. Infantile cortical hyperostosis

Answers overleaf

6. a. True
   b. False   This is commonly associated with mixed connective tissue disease
   c. True   And double-stranded DNA
   d. True   And C3 and C4 are low
   e. False   Only in 30%

7. a. True   Mainly in nutritional rickets
   b. True
   c. True   In most types of rickets
   d. True   In hypophosphataemic rickets
   e. True   In renal rickets

8. a. False   Craniotabes
   b. True
   c. True
   d. True
   e. False   Delayed closure of the fontanelle and absence of clavicle are the main features of craniocleidodysostosis

9. a. False
   b. True
   c. True
   d. False   Abnormal teeth
   e. False   This is a feature of thantophoric dwarfism

10. a. True
   b. False   Lytic
   c. True
   d. True
   e. True

11. Syndromes associated with absent radii include
   a. Fanconi's anaemia
   b. TAR
   c. Ellis–van-Creveld
   d. Holt–Oram
   e. Poland

12. HLA-B27 can be associated with the following conditions
   a. Inflammatory bowel disease
   b. Brucellosis
   c. Reiter's disease
   d. Psoriasis
   e. Ankylosing spondylitis

Answers overleaf

11. a. True   Pancytopenia and pigmented spots are other features

      b. True   Thrombocytopenia absent radius syndrome

      c. False   Post-axial polydactyly and ASD are features of this syndrome

      d. True   ASD is another feature of this syndrome

      e. False   This is associated with absence of the pectoralis major muscle and syndactyly

12. a. False   HLA-B27 is positive in inflammatory bowel disease

      b. False

      c. True

      d. False

      e. True

Eyes, ears, nose and throat

1. **The following statements relating to normal eyes are correct**
   a. The lateral rectus muscle is supplied by the abducens nerve
   b. The inferior oblique muscle is supplied by the trochlear nerve
   c. The aqueous humour has a low protein content
   d. The macula is the rod-free portion of the retina
   e. Cones are responsible for vision in dim light

2. **The following statements relating to the primary action of the eye muscles are correct**
   a. Superior oblique — depression
   b. Lateral rectus — adduction
   c. Superior rectus — inversion
   d. Inferior oblique — elevation
   e. Inferior rectus — eversion

3. **Aniridia**
   a. Has an autosomal dominant inheritance
   b. Is associated with Wilms' tumour in 50% of cases
   c. May cause glaucoma in more than half of patients
   d. Is commonly associated with corneal pannus
   e. May be associated with the Goldenhar syndrome

4. **Recognized risk factors which can cause central retinal vein occlusion include**
   a. Sickle cell anaemia
   b. Endocarditis
   c. Diabetes mellitus
   d. Hypermetropia
   e. Thalassaemia

5. **In Möbius' syndrome**
   a. Infantile feeding difficulties are common
   b. An expressionless face is a recognized feature
   c. Bilateral Vth cranial nerve palsies are characteristic
   d. The inheritance is autosomal dominant
   e. There may be associated deafness

Answers overleaf

1. a. True   This is the only muscle supplied by this nerve
   b. False   Superior oblique supplied by trochlear nerve. Oculomotor nerve supplies the other muscles of the eye
   c. True
   d. False   Fovea centralis is the rod-free portion of the retina
   e. False   Bright light

2. a. True   With secondary eversion and abduction
   b. False   Abduction
   c. False   Elevation with secondary abduction
   d. True   With secondary abduction and eversion
   e. False   Depression with secondary adduction and eversion

3. a. True   And usually bilateral
   b. False   In 20%
   c. True
   d. True
   e. False   Epibulbar colobomata is commonly associated with the Goldenhar syndrome

4. a. True   And central retinal artery occlusion
   b. True   Thrombo-embolic phenomena
   c. True   And diabetic retinopathy
   d. False
   e. False   Retinopathy may occur

5. a. True   Features of Möbius' syndrome include: congenital facial paresis and weakness of abduction of the eyes
   b. True
   c. False   VIIth cranial nerve palsies
   d. False   Sporadic
   e. True   Other associations include: pectoral and lingual muscle defects, ptosis, micrognathia, syndactyly and palatal and lingual palsies

6. **Large pupils are commonly associated with**
   a. Pontine haemorrhages
   b. The Holmes–Adie syndrome
   c. A IIIrd nerve palsy
   d. Horner's syndrome
   e. Tricyclic antidepressant poisoning

7. **Characteristic features of papilloedema include**
   a. Painful eye movements
   b. Loss of central vision
   c. Cupping of the optic disc
   d. Engorgement of the retinal veins as an early manifestation
   e. There may be an associated haemorrhage

8. **Causes of occulo-sympathetic paralysis (Horner's syndrome) include**
   a. Mid-brain lesions
   b. Neuroblastoma of the anterior mediastinum
   c. Posterior fossa tumours
   d. Brain-stem lesions
   e. Cervical ribs

9. **Dry eyes are a feature of**
   a. The Riley–Day syndrome
   b. Anhydrotic ectodermal dysplasia
   c. Dacrocystitis
   d. Glaucoma
   e. The Steven–Johnson syndrome

10. **Characteristic features of acute infective conjunctivitis include**
    a. Mucopurulent discharge
    b. Oedema of the eyes lids
    c. Cobblestone-like papules
    d. Itching
    e. Hyperaemia

Answers overleaf

6. a. False   Meiosis
    b. True   Absence of light and accommodation reflexes is another feature
    c. True   As well as trauma and atropine
    d. False   Unilateral ptosis, meiosis, enophthalmia, decreased facial sweating and flushing are features of Horner's syndrome
    e. True

7. a. False   Optic neuritis can cause this
    b. True
    c. False   Occurs with acute glaucoma
    d. True
    e. True

8. a. True   Occasionally familial
    b. False   Posterior mediastinal mass (neuroblastoma)
    c. False   Middle fossa tumours and cervical region tumours
    d. True
    e. True   And following thoracic surgery for congenital heart disease

9. a. True   Dysautonomia (failure to thrive, smooth tongue, fractured ribs and fever are features of this syndrome)
    b. True   X-linked recessive syndrome with fever and absence of sweating
    c. False   Associated with tears
    d. False
    e. True

10. a. True
    b. True   Common causes in neonates are gonococcal and chlamydia infections
    c. False   This is associated with vernal conjunctivitis
    d. False   This is a feature of allergic conjunctivitis
    e. True   And various degrees of ocular discomfort

11. Common causes of genetically-inherited cataracts include
   a. Toxoplasmosis
   b. Fabry disease
   c. Lowe's syndrome
   d. Insulin dependent diabetes mellitus (IDDM)
   e. Familial with autosomal dominant inheritance

12. Chorioretinitis is a feature of
   a. Toxocariasis
   b. Galactosaemia
   c. TORCH infection
   d. Tuberculosis
   e. Chloroquine ingestion

13. Causes of conductive hearing loss include
   a. Otosclerosis
   b. Foreign body
   c. Gentamicin therapy
   d. Cisplatinum therapy
   e. Perforation of the tympanic membrane

14. The common organisms causing acute otitis media include
   a. *Streptococcus pneumoniae*
   b. *Haemophilus influenzae*
   c. *Streptococcus pyogenes*
   d. *Staphylococcus aureus*
   e. *Branhamella catarrhalis*

15. Recognized complications following middle ear infection include
   a. Perforation of the tympanic membrane
   b. Brain abscess
   c. Pseudotumour cerebri
   d. Mastoiditis
   e. Facial paralysis

Answers overleaf

11. a. False   Congenital infection
    b. True   Galactosaemia, Wilson's disease and certain
                disorders of amino acid, calcium and copper
                metabolism can be associated with cataracts
    c. True
    d. False   Lens changes are uncommon
    e. True

12. a. True
    b. False   Cataract is a feature of galactosaemia
    c. True   Commonly with toxoplasmosis
    d. True   Complications due to chorioretinitis are retinal
                detachment and glaucoma
    e. False   Retinopathy

13. a. True
    b. True
    c. False   Sensorineural hearing loss
    d. False   Sensorineural hearing loss
    e. True

14. a. True   In 30%
    b. True   In 25%
    c. False   In 3% of cases only
    d. False   In 2% of cases only
    e. True   In 13%

15. a. True   And hearing loss
    b. True   Also extradural abscess and subdural empyema
    c. True   As well as lateral sinus thrombosis
    d. True
    e. True

16. Characteristic features of acute mastoiditis include
   a.   The pinna is displaced down and out
   b.   Purulent discharge
   c.   CT is a diagnostic investigation
   d.   Mastoidectomy should not be done
   e.   2nd and 3rd generation cephalosporins are an effective
        treatment

17. Causes of epistaxis include
   a.   Adenoidal hypertrophy
   b.   Sinusitis
   c.   Choanal atresia
   d.   Cystic fibrosis
   e.   Hypertension

Answers overleaf

16. a. True The primary clinical manifestations include:
swelling, redness and tenderness to touch of the
mastoid bone

 b. True Usually through a perforated tympanic membrane

 c. True May show hazyness or destruction of the mastoid
outline

 d. False Antibiotic therapy is the main treatment but
cortical mastoidectomy should also be done

 e. True

17. a. True

 b. True

 c. False Associated with difficulty in breathing

 d. True

 e. True

Community paediatrics

1. **The following radiological features may indicate non-accidental injuries (NAI) in children**
   a. Subperiosteal haemorrhage
   b. Metaphyseal-epiphyseal fracture
   c. Greenstick fracture
   d. Calcified old fractures at presentation
   e. Osteoporosis

2. **Criteria used to define screening procedures include**
   a. The incidence of the disease should be 1/2000 of the population
   b. A treatable condition
   c. The test is acceptable to the whole population
   d. The natural history of the condition is not important
   e. The test must be diagnostic of the condition

3. **Neonatal screening can be done for the following conditions**
   a. Deafness
   b. Down's syndrome
   c. Cataracts
   d. Congenital dislocation of the hip
   e. Phenylketonuria

4. **The chi-squared test is**
   a. Applied to a percentage
   b. Applied only to absolute numbers
   c. Never applied to proportion
   d. Equal to χ^2
   e. More sensitive than a student t-test

5. **Standard deviation (SD)**
   a. Is the square root of variance
   b. 1SD $\pm$ mean = 95% of values fall within that range
   c. Is the basis of the chi-squared test
   d. Is more than the standard error of the mean
   e. Is only of value for samples of small numbers

Answers overleaf

1. a. True
   b. True   This is called a bucket handle fracture
   c. False   Spiral fractures may be due to NAI
   d. True
   e. False

2. a. False
   b. True
   c. True
   d. False
   e. False

3. a. True
   b. True   This can be done prenatally and neonatally
   c. True
   d. True
   e. True   And hypothyroidism

4. a. False
   b. True
   c. True
   d. True
   e. False   Student t-test is more sensitive

5. a. True   Variance is the sum of the squares of the differences from the mean, divided by the number of observations minus one
   b. False   1 SD ± mean = 68%. 2SD means 95% of values fall within that range and 3SD gives 99.73% confidence limits
   c. False   Chi-squared compares frequency of a variable in two populations
   d. True
   e. False   SD is useful in the interpretation of data in terms of probability only if the population forms a normal distribution

6. **The following statements relating to enuresis are correct**
   a. It can be caused by infection
   b. Following normal micturation is psychogenic
   c. Urography and cystoscopy are usually done as the first line of investigation
   d. Enuretic children have a poor performance at school
   e. Waking the child repeatedly at night is a means of treatment

7. **The following statements relating to encopresis are correct**
   a. It is more common in males
   b. It is the passage of faeces in inappropriate places
   c. Social problems are more commonly associated with encopresis than enuresis
   d. Overflow incontinence indicates an organic defect
   e. Laxatives can be useful in its treatment

Answers overleaf

6. a. True
b. False
c. False
d. False
e. False

7. a. True
b. True
c. True
d. False
e. True

Poisoning

1. **Induced vomiting may be ineffective in the treatment of poisoning with**
   a. Anti-emetics
   b. Paracetamol
   c. Iron
   d. Atropine
   e. Phenothiazines

2. **Gastric lavage is still useful 12 hours after poisoning with**
   a. Salicylates
   b. Amphetamines
   c. Tricyclic anti-depressants
   d. Liquid paraffin
   e. Paraquat

3. **Recognized features of barbiturate poisoning include**
   a. Blisters
   b. Hypothermia
   c. Cerebral oedema
   d. Respiratory depression
   e. Tachycardia

4. **Characteristic features of salicylate poisoning in children include**
   a. Respiratory alkalosis
   b. Hyperventilation
   c. Hypothermia
   d. Hyperglycaemia
   e. Convulsions

5. **Lead encephalopathy is characterized by**
   a. Papilloedema
   b. Hypertension
   c. Ataxia
   d. Constipation
   e. Abdominal pain

Answers overleaf

169

1. a. True
    b. False
    c. False   Not if there is gastric erosion
    d. True   It has a cholinergic action
    e. True   It has a cholinergic action

2. a. True
    b. False   In the first 4 hours post ingestion
    c. True
    d. False   Not recommended
    e. False   Not recommended

3. a. True
    b. True
    c. True
    d. True
    e. False   Bradycardia

4. a. True
    b. True
    c. False   Usually hyperthermia
    d. False   Hypoglycaemia in children
    e. False

5. a. True   Headache, bradycardia and convulsions may
                occur
    b. False
    c. True   And personality problems
    d. False   Associated with chronic lead poisoning
    e. False   Associated with chronic lead poisoning

6. **Laboratory findings in chronic lead poisoning include**
a. Eosinophilic stippling .
b. Microcytic hypochromic anaemia
c. An increased urinary coproporphyrin
d. Increased blood levels of delta amino laevulinic acid
e. Proteinuria

7. **True or false**
a. Methanol poisoning causes severe metabolic alkalosis
b. Ethanol is the treatment for the methanol poisoning
c. Haemodialysis is effective in the treatment of phenothiazine poisoning
d. Carbon monoxide decreases the affinity of haemoglobin for oxygen
e. Amphetamines are never used in the management of anti-cholinergic poisoning

Answers overleaf

6. a. False   Basophilic stippling
    b. True
    c. True
    d. False   Usually increased in urine
    e. True   And amino-aciduria, glycosuria

7. a. False   Metabolites of methanol cause severe metabolic acidosis (formic acid and formaldehyde)
    b. True   Activated charcoal is contraindicated in the treatment of methanol poisoning
    c. False   Emesis or lavage, activated charcoal in large doses and benztropine for extrapyramidal side-effects
    d. True
    e. True